Understanding the Basics of Nutrition

ELIZABETH CARPENTER

UNDERSTANDING THE BASICS OF NUTRITION

2007

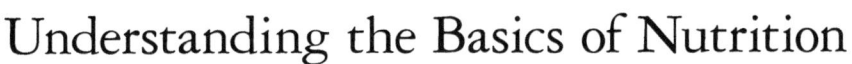

Understanding the Basics of Nutrition

Dedication

*To Those Who Desire To Keep The Temple—the Body—healthy,
Strong, And Fit For The Service Of God.*

TABLE OF CONTENTS

INTRODUCTION

At the start of every trip, I find myself in an airplane sitting next to a professional businessman. Usually, he inquires about the kind of work I do. I typically hope to find out more about the business he is in, but I smile and politely inform him that I am a nutrition and fitness consultant. Oh, they often reply, obviously not interested in the subject. However, sometimes they have some real questions about nutrition and want to clear up a few issues. When that happens, as it did on a recent flight, I listen sincerely and answer to the best of my abilities.

Just hearing the word nutrition conjures up all kinds of negative thoughts and vibes for most people. And any conversation quickly dwindles into excuses, as the beverage of choice and peanuts are passed out in mid-flight. But this time it was different. By the time the flight neared its end, and we found ourselves preparing to land, I knew that my having been seated next to this businessman was a blessing from God—for both him and myself.

I left the flight knowing that I needed to move forward with my desire to produce an educational nutrition book (regardless of the many diet and health books out there). My friend, the businessman, left knowing that he could change his unhealthy nutrition habits and begin eating healthy—even when traveling as he does due to working for a big corporation.

Living life—a truly abundant life—in every area, from a personal level to a spiritual level, seems to be a lost art. Many people appear to be just getting by, and tend to become satisfied with where they are. A reflection of this is how unhealthy most have become in the area of nutrition and caring for the body. Too many people suffer from serious health problems, are living lifestyles that will lead to health problems in the future, and are in bondage to food. Cancer, heart attacks, diabetes, obesity, and numerous other conditions affect millions of people each year, even though huge amounts of money are spent on medical care, drugs, and research. This situation has come about, in part, because so many have traveled down the wrong paths during the nutrition and fitness craze. Their lifestyles do not promote health, good nutrition, and the proper care of the body. Our society has become one of lazy people looking for the easy way out by cutting corners. Convenience is the key to living for most people—and the convenient, easy way is not often the best way.

As we go through this book, we will look at and discover how the body is meant to use food—to sustain it and allowed it to work at its optimum level—more or less from a textbook point of view. The purpose of this book is to educate, not to be another "diet" book that sits on the bookshelf collecting dust. We will learn more about nutrition, using helpful tips and examples found throughout this book, applying the knowledge we obtain to take care of our physical bodies. Simply by meeting our physical needs with the right kind of nutrients, we will free ourselves from the negative habits and thoughts we have toward food.

Many of my clients have said that once they were able to move beyond the bondage of food—to see food as the means of nourishing their bodies—it allowed them to live a healthier life. They were then able to see the deeper issues that needed to be addressed in other areas of their lives. Meeting the physical needs often provides the energy and motivation to deal with other issues at hand. Your reason for picking up this nutrition book—losing weight, gaining weight, controlling bad eating habits, getting well—does not matter. What matters is that you have come to a point where you realize there is more to life than merely surviving, like everyone around you. Realize that food is meant to nourish rather than harm you. Take the next step. Read this book and apply what you learn to your life now, knowing that in the end you will be in complete control of one area which tends to keep you from living a truly healthy and abundant life!

PART 1
An Overview of Nutrition

CHAPTER 1
About Nutrition

Food for Thought

Food is fuel for the body, and you burn the fuel at a rate (metabolism) that is unique for your body. Think of your body as a furnace that burns a set amount of fuel per day (energy requirements). If you put in too much fuel, the body will store the excess as fat. If you put in too little fuel, the body will burn stored reserves of fat and muscle. How much fuel you burn daily depends upon your body type (genetics), eating habits, age, activity, amount of lean muscle tissue, and so on.

Both food and the body are composed of nutrients and other essential materials. The six classes of nutrients are carbohydrates, proteins, fats, vitamins, minerals, and water. In the body, three of these nutrients— carbohydrates, proteins, and fats—are used to provide energy. In contrast, vitamins, minerals, and water do not yield any energy.

The body is designed to use the energy-yielding nutrients to fuel all its metabolic and physical activities. As the body metabolizes these nutrients, the bonds between their individual atoms break, which allows carbon and hydrogen atoms to combine with oxygen, yielding carbon dioxide and water for excretion. When the bonds between the carbon and hydrogen atoms break, they release energy. Some of this energy is given off as heat, but most of it is used as fuel throughout the whole body, as well as to send electrical impulses through the nerves and to synthesize body compounds.

If the body does not use these readily available nutrients to fuel metabolic and physical activities, it then stores these compounds in the body. For example, when a person eats in excess of energy needs, the body stores the excess as a small amount of glycogen and as much larger quantities of fat. Likewise, when food is not available to provide for energy needs, the body draws on its glycogen and fat stores for energy.

The amount of energy a food provides depends on how many carbohydrates, proteins, and fats it contains. This can be measured in calories—tiny units of energy called grams. When a nutrient is completely metabolized in the body, a gram of carbohydrate yields about 4 calories of energy. A gram of protein also yields 4 calories of energy and a gram of fat yields 9 calories of energy.

Technically speaking, nutrition is the science of how the body uses food. Healthful nutrition equals life. All living things need food and water to sustain life. You need healthful food—meaning food containing the proper nutrients—to live well. If you fail to eat and drink, you will die. But if you do not take caution, and you eat and drink to excess; you are setting yourself up for disease and illness, which leads to death as well.

Balance and moderation need to be applied when seeking to eat healthfully. In order to accomplish this, though, you need to know about why you eat what you eat and how the food affects the body.

An Overview of the Six Classes of Nutrients

Nutrients are chemical substances your body uses to build, maintain, and repair tissues, and to empower cells to send messages back and forth to conduct essential chemical reactions, such as the ones that make it possible for you to:

- Hear
- See
- Smell
- Taste
- Breathe
- Think
- Move

Food provides two different and distinct groups of nutrients:

- Macronutrients (macro means large)—carbohydrates, proteins, fats, and water
- Micronutrients (micro means small)—vitamins and minerals

The difference between each of these groups is the amount you need on a daily basis. Macronutrients are needed in larger quantities and micronutrients are needed in smaller quantities.

Carbohydrates

Carbohydrates supply the body with the energy it needs to function. Carbohydrates are mainly derived from plant foods, such as fruits, vegetables, whole grains, peas, and beans. Milk and milk products contain a significant amount of carbohydrates, and are the only foods which are from an animal source.

Carbohydrates are divided into two groups—complex carbohydrates and simple carbohydrates. Complex carbohydrates are made up of sugars, but the sugar molecules are strung together to form longer, more complex chains. Complex carbohydrates include fiber and starches. Foods that are richest in natural sources of complex carbohydrates include vegetables, whole grains, peas, and beans. Simple carbohydrates, sometimes referred to as simple sugars, are made up of shorter sugar molecule chains. Simple carbohydrates include fructose (fruit sugar), sucrose (table sugar), and lactose (milk sugar), as well as other sugars. Foods that are richest in natural sources of simple carbohydrates are fruits.

Carbohydrates are the main source of blood glucose, which is the major fuel for all cells in the body, and the only source of energy for the brain and red blood cells. Both complex and simple carbohydrates are converted into glucose, except for fiber, which cannot be digested. Glucose is used in the body to provide energy or is stored in the liver for future use. Again, when you consume more food than your body needs, a portion of the carbohydrate consumed may be stored as fat.

Fiber, a very important form of carbohydrate, is a necessary nutrient for the body. Commonly know as roughage, fiber is the part of plants that is resistant to the body's digestive enzymes. Only a small amount of fiber is digested or metabolized in the stomach or intestines. Most of it moves through the gastrointestinal tract and is eliminated from the body in the stool. Even though most fiber is not digested, it has several significant health benefits:

- Retains water, resulting in softer and bulkier stools that prevent constipation and hemorrhoids
- Reduces the risk of colon cancer, perhaps by speeding the rate at which stool passes through the intestine and by keeping the digestive tract clean
- Binds with certain substances that would generally result in the production of cholesterol, and eliminates these substances from the body

When choosing healthful carbohydrate sources, always select unrefined foods such as fruits, vegetables, peas, beans and whole grain products, as opposed to refined and processed foods such as sodas, desserts, candy, and sugar. Refined foods offer fewer, if any, vitamins and minerals that are important for overall health. When refined and processed foods are consumed as the majority of the diet or eaten in excess, especially over a period of time, it can lead to a number of health disorders, including diabetes.

Proteins

Protein is essential for growth and development. It provides the body with energy, and is needed for the manufacture of hormones, antibodies, enzymes, and tissues, as well as to help maintain proper acid-alkali balance in the body.

When protein is consumed, the body breaks it down into what are called amino acids, the building blocks of all protein. Proteins are divided into two groups—essential amino acids and nonessential amino acids. Essentials amino acids cannot be synthesized by the body and must be obtained from food. On the other hand, nonessential amino acids can be synthesized by the body from other amino acids.

Because of the importance of consuming proteins that provide all of the necessary amino acids, proteins are considered to belong to two different groups, depending on the amino acids (essential and nonessential) they provide. Complete proteins, which make up the first group, contain ample amounts of essential amino acids. These are found in meat, fish, poultry, cheese, eggs, and milk. Incomplete proteins, which make up the second group, contain only some of the essential amino acids. These proteins are found in a variety of foods, including whole grains, beans, and leafy green vegetables.

Although it is important to consume a wide array of amino acids, both essential and nonessential, it is not necessary to get them from meat, fish, poultry, and other complete-protein foods. A combination of incomplete-proteins foods can supply adequate amounts of all the essential amino acids. For example, although beans and brown rice are both rich in protein, each lacks one or more of the necessary amino acids. However, when combined with each other, or when either one is combined with any of a number of protein-rich foods, a complete protein is formed that is a high-quality substitute for meat.

Most people consume a diet high in protein. Although it is important to include protein in a healthful diet, you need to be aware of how much protein you are consuming. Eating too much protein may cause you to be at risk for high cholesterol or gout, a joint disorder. High-protein diets, such as the Atkins Diet, have also been implicated in kidney problems because of the extra effort the body must expend to process large amounts of protein. High-protein diets may also be high in fat and may lead to heart disease, if you are consuming high-fat protein sources. However, if you are eating a moderate amount of protein, you need to make sure you that you are getting enough.

When choosing healthful protein-rich sources, look for those that are minimally processed and handled, and are free of antibiotics and other chemicals.

Fats

Even though much attention has been focused on the need to reduce dietary fat, the body does need fat. During infancy and childhood, fat is necessary for normal brain development. However, after about two years of age, the body requires only small amounts of fat—much less than the average American diet provides. Throughout life, fat is essential in providing energy and supporting growth. Fat is the most concentrated source of energy available to the body. It must be noted, though, that excessive fat intake is a major contributing factor in obesity, high blood pressure, coronary heart disease, and colon cancer. It has been linked to a number of other disorders as well.

Fats are composed of building blocks called fatty acids. There are three major categories of fatty acids—saturated, polyunsaturated, and monosaturated. These classifications are based on the number of hydrogen atoms in the chemical makeup of a given molecule of fatty acid.

The liver uses saturated fats to manufacture cholesterol. Excessive dietary intake of saturated fats can significantly raise the blood cholesterol level, especially the level of low-density lipoproteins (LDL), known as "bad cholesterol." Saturated fats can be found in the following foods:

- Animal products: fatty cuts of meats like beef, veal, lamb, pork and ham. A fatty cut is one that has a lot of marbling in the meat itself. This is the saturated fat in the meat.

- Dairy products: whole milk, cream, and whole fat cheeses.
- Vegetable products: coconut oil, palm kernel oil, and vegetable shortening.

Saturated fats should be limited to about 10 percent of the overall diet.

Unlike saturated fats, polyunsaturated fats may actually lower the total blood cholesterol level. However, the intake of high amounts of polyunsaturated fats has a tendency to reduce high-density lipoproteins (HDL), known as "good cholesterol." Polyunsaturated fats can be found in the following foods:

- Corn
- Soybeans
- Safflower and sunflower oils
- Certain fish oils

Polyunsaturated fats should be limited to about 10 percent of the overall diet.

It appears that monosaturated fats reduce the blood levels of LDL without affecting the blood levels of HDL in any way.

Monosaturated fats can be found in the following foods:

- Vegetables
- Nuts
- Nut oil
- Olive and canola oil

Monosaturated fats should be limited to about 10-15 percent of the overall diet.

Most foods—including plant-derived foods—contain a combination of all three types of fatty acids. Thus, a fat or oil is considered "saturated" when it is composed primarily of saturated fatty acids, or "polyunsaturated" when it is composed primarily of polyunsaturated fatty acids, and so on.

Another component to consider in the topic of fats is trans-fatty acids. This form of fatty acids occurs when polyunsaturated oils are altered through hydrogenation, a process used to harden liquid vegetable oils into solid foods like margarine and shortening. Nowadays, hydrogenated oils are put into a lot of products we consume. It is important to be aware of the products that contain hydrogenated oils and not to consume a lot of these products. It has been found that trans-fatty acids do have a negative effect on the blood cholesterol levels.

When choosing healthful fat sources, you should look for foods with low levels of saturated fats and trans-fatty acids.

Water

The body is made up of about 75 percent of water. Water is an essential nutrient that is involved in every function of the body. It helps to transport nutrients and waste products in and out of the cells. It is required for all digestive, absorptive, circulatory, and excretory functions. It is used for the utilization of water-soluble vitamins. It also is needed for keeping the body's temperature at a suitable level. The body should stay well hydrated in order to maintain good health. Drinking enough water throughout each day—at least eight 8-ounce glasses—will accomplish this. It should be noted that some people may require more water than others; that is fine, as long as you get the amount your body needs.

Vitamins and Minerals

Like carbohydrates, proteins, fats, and water, vitamins and minerals are essential to life. They are therefore considered nutrients, but are needed in relatively small amounts compared to the four basic nutrients.

Vitamins contribute to good health by regulating the metabolism and assisting the biochemical processes that release energy from digested food.

Some of these vitamins are water soluble and some are fat soluble. Water-soluble vitamins must be taken into the body daily, because they cannot be stored. They are excreted within fours hours to one day. These include vitamin C and the B-complex vitamins. Fat-soluble vitamins are retained in the body for longer periods of time, because they are stored in the body's fatty tissue and liver. These include vitamins A, D, E, and K. Both forms of vitamins are needed and are used by the body for proper function.

Minerals are needed for the proper composition of body fluids, the formation of blood and bone, the maintenance of healthy nerve function, muscle tone of the body, and the cardiovascular system. Because all enzyme activity involves minerals, they are needed for the proper utilization of vitamins and other nutrients.

Nutritionally, minerals are divided into two groups: bulk minerals and trace minerals. Bulk minerals include calcium, magnesium, sodium, potassium, and phosphorus. These are needed in greater amounts than trace minerals. Nevertheless, traces minerals are still of great importance. Trace minerals include boron, chromium, copper, germanium, iodine, iron, manganese, molybdenum, selenium, silicon, sulfur, vanadium, and zinc.

Because vitamins and minerals are so necessary for health, the U.S. Food and Drug Administration (FDA) has recommended consumption levels for vitamins and minerals called Reference Daily Intake (RDIs). Although these allowances are safe (i.e., they will not cause toxicity), they should be varied according to a person's size and weight. People who are active and exercise, under great stress, on restricted diets, mentally or physically ill, taking oral contraceptives, on medication, recovering from surgery, and those who smoke or consume large amounts of alcoholic beverages all need various amounts of vitamins and minerals.

Nutrients in Foods and in the Body

The body is able to derive all the energy, structural materials, and regulating agents that it needs from the foods consumed. The foods you consume are made up of the six classifications of nutrients—substances used for the growth, maintenance, and repair of the body. A complete chemical analysis of the body would prove that it is made up of materials similar to those found in foods. For example, a healthy 150-lb. person contains about 90 lbs. of water and about 30 lbs. of fat. The other 30 lbs. consist of mostly compounds containing carbohydrate, protein, and the major minerals of the bones. Vitamins and the other minerals constitute a fraction of a pound.

The body has the ability to make some nutrients, and it can make these nutrients in sufficient quantities to meet its needs. But it cannot make all of them, so it is necessary to obtain these nutrients from foods. These are referred to as essential nutrients. Foods contain mostly essential nutrients, but they provide other compounds as well—alcohols, phytochemicals, pigments, additives, and others. Some are beneficial, neutral, and few are found to be harmful. These compounds do not fit within the six classes of nutrients and are referred to as non-nutrients.

The Energy-Yielding Nutrients

In the body, carbohydrates, proteins, and fats can be used to provide energy. In contrast, vitamins, minerals, and water are not energy-yielding, and are not used by the body to provide energy.

The energy released from carbohydrates, proteins, and fats is measured in calories—tiny units of energy. To better understand calculations, energy is expressed in 1000-calorie metric units known as kilocalories (shortened to kcalories, but commonly referred to as calories). When you read in nutrition books or magazines that an apple provides 100 calories, understand that it means 100 kcalories. A kcalorie is not a constituent of foods; it is a measure of potential energy in foods. Therefore, to speak of kcalories in an apple is technically incorrect, just as to speak of inches in a person is incorrect. It is correct to speak of the energy a food provides, just as it is of the height of a person.

The amount of energy a food supplies depends on the amount of carbohydrates, proteins, and fats it contains. Again, a gram of carbohydrate yields about 4 calories of energy. A gram of protein also yields 4 calories of energy and a gram of fat yields 9 calories of energy. Another substance that is metabolized by the body and is energy-yielding is alcohol. Alcohol is not considered a nutrient because it interferes with proper growth, maintenance, and repair of the body, but it does yield energy—about 7 calories of energy when metabolized by the body.

The body uses the energy-yielding nutrients to fuel all its functions and activities. As the body metabolizes these nutrients, the bonds between their individual atoms break, which allows carbon and hydrogen atoms to combine with oxygen, yielding carbon dioxide and water for excretion. When the bonds between the carbon and hydrogen atoms break, they release energy. Some of this energy is given off as heat, but most of it is used as fuel throughout the whole body, as well as to send electrical impulses through the nerves and to synthesize body compounds. The energy used from food supports every activity, from quiet thought to long-distance running.

If the body does not use these readily available nutrients, it then stores these compounds in the body. For example, when a person eats in excess of energy needs, the body stores this (such as body fat) for use when fresh energy supplies run low. Likewise, when food is not available to provide for energy needs, the body draws on its stores (such as body fat and muscle) for energy.

When consumed in excess of energy need, alcohol can be converted to body fat and stored. Alcohol is apart of most individual's diet nowadays, and the harm it does—when consumed in excess—extends far beyond the problems of body fat.

In addition to providing energy, carbohydrates, proteins, and fats provide the raw materials for building the body's tissues and regulating its many functions. For example, protein's role as a fuel source is relatively minor compared with both of the other two nutrients and their roles. Proteins are found in structures such as the muscles and skin, and they help to regulate functions such as digestion and energy metabolism.

Chemical Reactions in the Body

How do you obtain energy from foods? The process occurs when the body releases energy from the chemical bonds in the nutrients it is using as fuel. As the bonds break, they release energy in a controlled version of the process by which wood burns as fuel for a fire. Both wood and food have the potential to provide energy. When wood burns in the presence of oxygen, it generates heat and light (energy), steam (water), and some carbon dioxide and ash (waste). Likewise, during the body's metabolism, energy, water, and carbon dioxide are released. All of these, and other chemical reactions that go on in living cells, are collectively known as metabolism. Energy metabolism includes all the ways the body obtains and spends energy from food.

The groundwork of metabolism starts during digestion, when the body breaks down the three energy-yielding nutrients—carbohydrates, proteins, and fats—into four basic units, which are then able to be absorbed into the bloodstream. The four basic units along with their major sources are:

- From carbohydrates—glucose
- From proteins—amino acids
- From fats—glycerol and fatty acids

Building Up and Breaking Down

The cells in the body can use the basic units of energy-yielding nutrients to build compounds. For instance, glucose molecules may be joined together to make glycogen chains; amino acids may be linked together to make proteins; glycerol and fatty acids may be assembled into triglycerides. Each of these reactions starts with small, simple compounds and uses them as building blocks to form larger, more complex structures. Such reactions involve doing work and thus require energy. The building up of body compounds is known as anabolism—a reaction in which small molecules are put together to form larger molecules.

The breaking down of body compounds is known as catabolism—a reaction in which large molecules are broken down into smaller molecules. Catabolism reactions include the breakdown of glycogen to glucose, of proteins to amino acids, and of triglycerides to glycerol and fatty acids. When the body is in need of energy, it breaks down any or all of these four basic units into even smaller units.

When a chemical bond breaks, energy is released as heat, can be captured in another chemical bond, or both. Frequently, as one compound is broken apart, some energy is released as heat and some is used to put together another compound. Such reactions, in which the compound is broken and one compound provides energy for the building of another, are known as coupled reactions—a pair of chemical reactions where energy released from the breakdown of one compound is used to create a bond in the formation of another compound.

Transferring of Energy in Reactions

The energy released during catabolism is often captured by passing molecules which tend to easily transfer that energy to other compounds. These molecules are known as ATP (adenosine triphosphate)—a common high-energy compound composed of purine (adenine), a sugar (ribose), and three phosphate groups.

ATP is one of the body's quick-energy molecules and its name indicates that it contains three phosphate groups. The energy bond between each phosphate group is greater than the energy in most other chemical bonds. When energy is needed, a hydrolysis reaction breaks these high-energy bonds by splitting off one or two phosphate groups and releases their energy. These reactions are coupled to other reactions which use that energy as well. Therefore, the body uses ATP to transfer the energy produced during catabolic reactions to power its anabolic reactions.

Metabolic reactions are going on all the time within the body's cells. The type and extent of metabolic activity varies depending on the kind of cell, but of all the body's cells, the liver cells are the most adaptable and metabolically active.

Nearly all metabolic reactions require the assistance of enzymes. Enzyme helpers are known as coenzymes—small organic molecules that work with enzymes to facilitate the enzymes' activities. The relationship between enzymes and coenzymes differ, but one thing is certain: an enzyme cannot function without its coenzyme. For example, some of the B vitamins serve as coenzymes to the enzymes that release energy from glucose, amino acids, glycerol, and fatty acids. These B vitamin coenzymes come alongside the metabolic pathways and help to keep the disassembly lines moving, so to speak.

During digestion, the energy-yielding nutrients—carbohydrates, proteins, and fats—are broken down into glucose, amino acids, glycerol, and fatty acids. Aided by enzymes and coenzymes, the cells use these products of digestion to build more complex compounds (anabolism) or break them down even further to release energy (catabolism). The energy released during catabolism is often taken in by high-energy compounds such as ATP.

Breaking Down the Nutrients for Energy

It is now time to enter a cell and follow the various paths that glucose, amino acids, glycerol, and fatty acids take to yield energy. Each compound starts down a different path, but they all reach a common destination. What happens to these compounds inside cells can best be understood by starting with the breakdown of glucose.

Glucose

When talking about the breaking down of glucose, two new names appear—pyruvate (a 3-carbon compound that plays a key role in energy metabolism) and acetyl CoA (a 2-carbon compound with a coenzyme attached). All compounds that are able to be converted to pyruvate can be used to make glucose. However, the compounds that are converted directly to acetyl CoA cannot make glucose.

The first pathway glucose takes is called glycolysis—the metabolic breakdown of glucose to pyruvate. As the process of glucose yielding energy proceeds, the 6-carbon glucose is split in half, forming two 3-carbon compounds. The 3-carbon compounds continue down the pathway until they are converted to pyruvate. The net yield of one glucose molecule is two pyruvate molecules. If the glucose molecule continues to break down, both pyruvate molecules will release much of their energy to form ATP molecules, and some of their energy as heat.

A cell is able to make glucose again from pyruvate in a process similar to the reversal of glycolysis. Making glucose merely requires energy and a few different enzymes. Therefore, glucose is retrievable from pyruvate.

When the splitting process of glucose to pyruvate starts, the cell uses little energy. But then it produces more energy than it had to be supplied with initially. At this point no oxygen has been required so far, which means glycolysis is an anaerobic pathway. More energy can be released when taking the pyruvate through additional metabolic reactions, but oxygen is needed for these reactions, which are aerobic. With adequate oxygen, pyruvate molecules enter the mitochondria of the cell where they will be converted to acetyl CoA.

Once the cell needs energy and oxygen is available, it eliminates a carbon group from the 3-carbon pyruvate to produce a 2-carbon compound, which attaches to a molecule of CoA and becomes acetyl CoA. The carbon group from pyruvate becomes carbon dioxide, which is released into the bloodstream, circulated to the lungs, and breathed out.

On the other hand, when less oxygen is available, pyruvate is converted to lactic acid—a 3-carbon compound produced from pyruvate during anaerobic metabolism. This anaerobic reaction occurs to some degree even when the body is at rest, but it increases dramatically during high-intensity exercise. This happens whenever exertion exceeds the capacity of the heart and lungs to deliver oxygen to and clear carbon dioxide from the muscles. When oxygen availability and carbon dioxide clearance is limited, lactic acid builds up in the muscles, causing a burning sensation and fatigue. To relieve the burning sensation, the muscles must be relaxed frequently so that the circulating blood can transport the lactic acid away to the liver. The liver is able to convert lactic acid to glucose in what is referred to as the Cori cycle—the path from muscle glycogen to glucose to pyruvate to lactic acid (which travels to the liver) to glucose (which is able to travel back to the muscle) to glycogen. Muscle cells do not have the necessary enzyme to recycle lactic acid to glucose.

The step from pyruvate to acetyl CoA is metabolically irreversible. A cell cannot regain the shed carbons from the carbon dioxide to remake pyruvate, and then back to glucose.

Acetyl CoA may take different metabolic paths, depending on the cell's need. If the cell needs energy, acetyl CoA may produce this through a series of reactions referred to as the TCA (Tricarboxylic Acid) cycle—a series of metabolic reactions that break down molecules of acetyl CoA to carbon dioxide and hydrogen atoms; and the ETC (Electron Transport Chain)—the final pathway in energy metabolism where the electrons from hydrogen are passed to oxygen and where the energy released is trapped in the bonds of ATP. These reactions convert the 2-carbon acetyl CoA to 2-carbon dioxide molecules and free up its coenzyme (CoA) to be reused. During this process, much more energy is released than during glycolysis.

If energy is not needed, acetyl CoA will not enter into the TCA cycle, but instead will be used to make fatty acids. This is why the consumption of carbohydrates, and even protein or fat in excess of the body's needs, can add to fat stores.

In summary, the main steps in the catabolism of glucose are as follows:

Glucose—> Pyruvate—> Acetyl CoA—> Carbon Dioxide

Amino Acids

Amino acids are deaminated (they lose their nitrogen containing amino group), and then they are catabolized in a variety of ways. A number of amino acids can be converted to pyruvate, others are converted to acetyl CoA, and still others enter the TCA cycle directly as compounds other than acetyl CoA.

Amino acids that are used to make pyruvate can provide glucose, while those used to make acetyl CoA can provide additional energy or make body fat but cannot make glucose. Amino acids entering the TCA cycle directly can continue in the cycle and generate energy; otherwise, they can generate glucose. Therefore, protein is a fairly good source of glucose when carbohydrates are not available.

A major part of understanding these metabolic pathways of protein is learning which fuels can be converted to glucose and which cannot. The parts of protein that can be converted to pyruvate can provide glucose for the body, whereas the parts that are converted to acetyl CoA cannot provide glucose, but can readily provide fat. The body must have glucose to fuel the activities of the central nervous system and red blood cells. If it does not obtain glucose from food, the body will consume its own lean tissue to provide the protein to make glucose. To keep this from happening, you need to supply fuels that provide glucose—primary carbohydrates. If you feed your body only fat, which delivers mostly acetyl CoA, you put your body in the position of having to break down protein tissue to make glucose. If you fuel your body with only protein, you put your body in the position of having to convert protein to glucose. Without a doubt, the best diet supplies a balance of carbohydrates, proteins, and fats.

Once amino acids have been converted to acetyl CoA, if energy is not needed, fatty acids are made and stored as triglycerides in adipose tissue (the body's fat tissue, consisting of masses of fat-storing cells). Thus, protein can also add to fat stores if eaten in excess. Those who eat large portions of meat and other protein-rich foods may wonder why they have weight problems. Not only does the fat in those foods lead to fat storage, but the protein can, too, when intake exceeds energy needs.

Back to the deamination of amino acids: when amino acids are metabolized for energy or used to make fat, they must be deaminated first. Two products result from deamination. One is the carbon structure without its amino group often referred to as keto acid—an organic acid that contains a carbonyl group. The other product is referred to as ammonia—a compound with the chemical formula of NH_3. Ammonia is a base, and if the body produces larger amounts than it can handle, the blood's acid-base balance becomes upset.

The next step is referred to as transamination—the transfer of an amino acid to a keto acid, producing a new nonessential amino acid and a new keto acid. By transferring an amino group from one amino acid to its corresponding keto acid, cells can make a new amino acid and a new keto acid. Through many such transamination reactions, involving many different keto acids, the liver cells are able to synthesize the nonessential amino acids. Remember, only some amino acids are essential; the others can be made in the body, if given a source of nitrogen.

The liver continuously produces small amounts of ammonia during deamination reactions. Some of this ammonia provides nitrogen needed for the synthesis of nonessential amino acids. The liver combines any remaining ammonia with carbon dioxide to make what is known as urea—the principal nitrogen excretion product of metabolism. Two ammonia fragments are combined with carbon dioxide to form urea.

Once the liver cells release the urea into the bloodstream, it circulates until it passes through the kidneys. The kidneys remove the urea from the blood for excretion in the urine. The liver efficiently captures all the ammonia, makes urea from it, and releases the urea into the bloodstream;

then the kidneys clear all the urea from the blood. This process allows for easy diagnosis of diseases of both the liver and kidneys. If the liver or kidneys are not functioning properly, blood ammonia levels will be high.

Urea is the body's principal means of excreting unused nitrogen, and the amount produced increases with protein intake. To keep urea levels in balance in the body, it is important to consume an appropriate amount of water. A person who regularly consumes a high-protein diet (100 grams a day or more) must drink more water than usual. Without the extra water, the person risks an accumulation of urea in the blood.

In summary, the body is able to use some amino acids to produce glucose, while others can be used to generate energy or to be stored as body fat. Before an amino acid enters one of the metabolic pathways, its nitrogen containing amino group must be removed through the process of deamination. A number of nitrogen's may be used to make nonessential amino acids and other nitrogen containing compounds. The rest are then cleared from the body through urea synthesis in the liver and excretion in the kidneys.

Glycerol and Fatty Acids

Once the breakdown of glucose is understood, protein and fat breakdown are easily learned, for all three share a common metabolic pathway. Remember that triglycerides are broken down to glycerol and fatty acids. Glycerol is easily converted to another 3-carbon compound to form pyruvate and acetyl CoA, and then to make carbon dioxide. Unlike glycerol, fatty acids are taken apart 2 carbons at a time, in a series of aerobic reactions referred to as fatty acid oxidation—the metabolic breakdown of fatty acids to acetyl CoA.

Only a little energy is released each time a 2-carbon fragment breaks off from a fatty acid during oxidation, but nearly three times as much energy is released when these 2-carbon units of acetyl CoA enter the TCA cycle. If the cell does not need energy, the acetyl CoA molecules will combine with each other to make body fat, in the same way acetyl CoA produced from excess carbohydrates does.

Cells are able to make glucose from pyruvate and other 3-carbon compounds, such as glycerol, but they cannot make glucose from the 2-carbon fragments of fatty acids. The significance of this is that fat, for the most part, is unable to provide energy for red blood cells, the brain, or the nervous system, all of which require glucose as their fuel source.

Remember, almost all dietary fats are triglycerides, and triglycerides contain only one small molecule of glycerol with three fatty acids. Therefore, fat is an insignificant source of glucose. Roughly 95 percent of fat cannot be converted to glucose.

In summary, the body is able to convert the small glycerol portion of a triglyceride to either pyruvate (and then glucose) or acetyl CoA. The fatty acid of a triglyceride, on the other hand, is unable to make glucose, but this acid can provide acetyl CoA. From either source, acetyl CoA may then enter the TCA cycle to produce energy, or combine with the other molecules of acetyl CoA to make body fat.

Food Choices

People decide what to eat and when to eat in highly personal ways, often based on behavioral or social motives more than on awareness of nutrition or its importance to health. Luckily, many different food choices can be healthy ones, but nutrition awareness always helps to make them so. The following are reasons that influence food choices:

- Personal Preference
- Habit
- Ethnic Heritage or Tradition
- Social Interactions
- Availability, Convenience, and Economy
- Positive and Negative Associations
- Emotional Comfort
- Values
- Weight and Body Image
- Nutritional Values

Several times a day, you make food choices that influence your body's health or lack of it. Each day's choices may benefit or harm your health, and when these choices are repeated over time, the rewards or consequences add up. That being the case, cultivating good eating habits and healthful food choices can and will bring health benefits, both now and in the years to come. Conversely, carelessness in eating habits and food choices will only lead to prevalent chronic diseases and other health problems later in life. Of course, some people will die young no matter what choices they make with regard to their eating habits and overall health, and others will live long lives despite making poor choices. Still, whatever your reasons, the food choices you make each day will affect—either benefit or impair—your overall health. Individual food selections neither make nor break a diet's healthfulness, but a balance of food selected over time can make a difference in the body's overall health.

Dietary Reference Intake

Defining the amounts of energy, nutrients, and other dietary factors that best support overall health is a large task. Nutrition experts have produced a set of energy and nutrient standards. These standards are revised periodically as new evidence becomes available or needs are updated. The current revisions work to maintain the original goal of protecting against nutrient deficiencies, but given the wealth of research now connecting diet and health, that goal has been expanded to include supporting optimal activities within the body and preventing chronic diseases.

With this aim in mind, a major revision of nutrient recommendations was implemented. These recommendations are referred to as the Dietary Reference Intake (DRI), and they are the collaborative efforts of researchers in both the United States and Canada. The DRI is a set of guidelines for dietary nutrient intake designed to promote the health of people in the United States and Canada. These values are used for planning and assessing diets, and include:

- Estimated Average Requirements (EAR)
- Recommended Daily Intake (RDI)
- Adequate Intakes (AI)
- Tolerable Upper Intake Levels (UL)

The Dietary Reference Intake committee consists of highly qualified scientists who base their estimates of nutrient needs on careful examination and explanation of scientific evidence.

The committee reviews countless research studies to establish the requirement for a nutrient—how much is needed in the diet. A different measure for each nutrient is selected, based on its roles both in performing activities in the body and in reducing disease risk. With this information, the estimated average requirement is determined. The estimated average requirement is the amount of a nutrient that will maintain a specific biochemical or physiological function in half the people of a given age and gender group. In other words, it is used to determine the nutrient amount that appears sufficient to maintain a specific body function in men and women of differing ages. An examination of all available data reveals that each person's body is unique and has its own set of requirements.

The average daily amount of a nutrient considered adequate to meet the known nutrient needs of practically all healthy people is referred to as the Recommended Daily Intake (RDA). The committee must also decide what intake to recommend for all healthy individuals in general. These recommendations should be set high enough above the estimated average requirement in order to meet the needs of most healthy people. Nearly everyone would be covered if they met this dietary goal. Relatively few people's requirements would exceed these recommendations, and even then, they would not exceed by very much. In contrast to the recommendations for nutrients, the value set for energy needs is not as generous. Instead, it is set at the mean of the population's estimated requirements, representing the average needs of any one individual. Only enough energy is needed to sustain a healthy and active life, but consuming too many calories (energy) can lead to obesity and other major health problems.

For some nutrients, there is insufficient data or scientific evidence to determine an Estimated Average Requirement, which is needed to set the Recommended Dietary Allowance. In cases such as these, the committee establishes what is referred to as an Adequate Intake (AI)—the average amount of a nutrient that appears sufficient to maintain a specified criterion. An Adequate Intake reflects the average amount of a nutrient that a group of healthy people consume. Like the Recommended Dietary Allowances, the Adequate Intake may be used by individuals as nutrient goals.

The recommended intakes for nutrients are generous, and though they do not always cover every individual for every nutrient, they probably should not be exceeded, as people's tolerances for high doses of nutrients vary. Above the recommended intake is what is referred to as the Tolerable Upper Intake Level (UL)—the maximum amount of a nutrient that appears safe for most healthy people, and beyond which there is an increased risk of adverse health effects. These upper levels are particularly useful in safeguarding against consuming too much of any nutrient, vitamin or mineral, which is likely to occur when using supplements or eating fortified foods regularly.

Although the intent of nutrient recommendations may seem simple enough, they are the subject of much misunderstanding. The following points should help put them in perspective:

- Estimates of adequate energy and nutrient intakes apply to healthy individuals. They do not apply to undernourished people, or to those with medical problems which may require supplemented or restricted intakes.

- These recommendations include a generous margin of safety; they are not minimum requirements, nor are they necessarily optimal intakes for all individuals.

- Recommendations apply to average daily intakes. The length of time over which an individual's intake can deviate from the average without risk of deficiency or overdose varies for each nutrient, depending on the body's use and storage of the nutrient. Trying to meet recommendations for every nutrient every day is difficult and unnecessary.

- Most nutrient goals are intended to be met through healthful diets composed of a variety of foods, when possible. Foods contain a mixture of nutrients and non-nutrients, and deliver more than just those nutrients covered by the recommendations. Excess intakes of vitamins and minerals are unlikely when their sources are foods rather than supplements.

In summary, the Dietary Reference Intakes (DRI) are a set of four nutrient intake values that can be used to plan and evaluate healthful diets for healthy individuals. The estimated average requirement defines the amount of a nutrient that supports a specific function in the body. The Recommended Dietary Allowance (RDA) is based on the estimated average requirement, and establishes a goal for dietary intake that will meet the needs of nearly all healthy individuals. An Adequate Intake (AI) serves a similar purpose when a Recommended Dietary Allowance cannot be determined. The Tolerable Upper Intake Level (UL) establishes the highest amount that appears safe for regular consumption.

The key to sustaining nutritional health is to understand how the body functions and how it uses nutrients to run all of its systems. When the body operates as it was designed to, you will be able to maintain your overall health and fitness in order to live well and function properly.

CHAPTER 2
About Carbohydrates

When people sit quietly and read an intriguing novel, they are completely unaware that within their brain cells, billions of glucose molecules are splitting each and every second to supply the energy that allows them to read. Glucose provides nearly all of the energy the brain uses daily. Similarly, marathon runners reaching the finish line seldom celebrate the fact that glycogen fueled their muscles and allowed them to finish the race. Together, glucose and its storage form, glycogen, provide about half of all the energy that muscles and other body tissues use.

People do not eat glucose and glycogen directly, but they consume foods that are rich in carbohydrates. Once you have consumed the carbohydrate food, the body converts the carbohydrates into glucose for immediate energy and into glycogen for reserve energy.

Many mistakenly think that carbohydrates are "fattening" and seek to avoid them altogether. However, all unrefined plant foods—whole grains, vegetables, legumes, and fruits—provide ample healthful carbohydrate and fiber without added processed ingredients or fat.

The Breakdown of Carbohydrates

Carbohydrates are broken down into two main categories—simple carbohydrates (sugars) and complex carbohydrates (starches and fibers). Simple carbohydrates are made up of monosaccharides (single sugars) and disaccharides (sugars composed of pairs of monosaccharides). Complex carbohydrates are made up of only polysaccharides (large molecules composed of chains of monosaccharides).

Simple Carbohydrates
Monosaccharides

The three monosaccharides important in nutrition have the same number and types of atoms, but they differ in arrangement. The chemical differences account for the differing sweetness of each monosaccharide. A pinch of galactose on the tongue hardly tastes sweet at all, and purified glucose gives only a mildly sweet flavor. But fructose is as intensely sweet as honey.

Galactose is rarely seen occurring in nature because it binds with glucose to form the sugar in milk. Galactose has the same numbers and types of atoms as glucose and fructose, but in a different arrangement form.

Glucose, commonly known as blood sugar, serves as an essential energy source for all the body's activities, and it is very significant to nutrition. Glucose is one of the two sugars in every disaccharide, and is the unit from which the polysaccharides are made almost entirely.

Fructose is the sweetest of all the three sugars. It contains the same chemical makeup as glucose, but the arrangement form is slightly different. The arrangement of the atoms in fructose causes the taste buds on the tongue to taste a sweet sensation, which gives the sweet taste in the mouth. Fructose occurs naturally in fruits and honey; other sources are found in products such as soft drinks, cereals, and desserts that have been sweetened with high-fructose corn syrup.

Disaccharides

The disaccharides are pairs of the three monosaccharides just discussed. In order to make a disaccharide, a chemical reaction known as condensation takes place—in which two reactants combine to yield a larger product. To break a disaccharide in half, hydrolysis has to take place. This is when a molecule of water splits to provide the resulting monosaccharides. Such reactions commonly occur during digestion.

The three disaccharides that are important in nutrition are maltose—a disaccharide composed of two glucose units, sometimes known as malt sugar; sucrose—a disaccharide composed of glucose and fructose, commonly known as table sugar; and lactose—a disaccharide composed of glucose and galactose, commonly known as milk sugar.

Maltose is composed of two glucose units and is produced whenever a starch is broken down, such as during the digestion of carbohydrates in the body. It also happens during the fermentation process that yields alcohol. Maltose is only a minor component of a few foods.

Sucrose is formed from the combination of glucose and fructose. Since the fructose is sweet to the taste buds, sucrose tastes sweet as well, and accounts for some of the natural sweetness of fruits, vegetables, and grains. To make table sugar, sucrose is refined from the juices of sugar cane and sugar beets, and then it is granulated. Depending on the degree to which it is refined, the sugar becomes brown, white, or powdered sugar.

Lactose is the combination of glucose and galactose. It is known as milk sugar, and contributes to about 5 percent of the milk's weight.

In summary, the six simple carbohydrates (sugar) are important in nutrition. The three monosaccharides (galactose, glucose, and fructose) all have the same chemical makeup, but their structures differ. The three disaccharides (maltose, sucrose, and lactose) are pairs of monosaccharides, each containing a glucose paired with one of three monosaccharides. The sugars are primarily derived from plants, except for lactose and its component, galactose, which come from milk and milk products. Again, two monosaccharides can be linked together by a condensation reaction to form a disaccharide and water. A disaccharide, in turn, can be broken into its two monosaccharides by a hydrolysis reaction using water.

Complex Carbohydrates

Complex carbohydrates contain many glucose units and, in some cases, a few other monosaccharides, which, as discussed earlier, are a simple carbohydrate. The complex carbohydrate that contains a few other monosaccharides strung together is known as a polysaccharide—a compound of many monosaccharides linked together. Three polysaccharides are important in nutrition: glycogen, starches, and fibers.

Glycogen is a storage form of energy in the body. Both glycogen and starch are built of glucose units, but they are linked together differently. Fibers are composed of a variety of monosaccharides and other carbohydrates, and they will be explored later.

Glycogen

Glycogen is found in a limited amount of meat and not in plants at all. It is an animal polysaccharide composed of glucose. It is manufactured and stored in the liver and muscles as a storage form of glucose. Glycogen is not a significant food source of carbohydrate and is not counted as one of the complex carbohydrates in food. However, it does perform an important process in the body. The body stores much of its glucose as glycogen. This arrangement permits rapid hydrolysis. When the message to release energy arrives at the storage sites in the liver or muscle cells, enzymes respond by attacking all the many branches of each glycogen simultaneously, making a surge of glucose available in the blood.

Starches

Just as the body stores glucose as glycogen, plant cells store glucose as starches—long branched or un-branched chains of hundreds or thousands of glucose molecules linked together—which come from plant polysaccharides composed of glucose.

All starchy foods are derived from plants, and grains are the richest food source of starches. The main supply of starches includes grains, legumes, and tubers such as potatoes, yams, and cassava.

Fiber

Fibers are the structural parts of plants and are found in all plant-derived foods such as vegetables, fruits, grains, and legumes. Most fibers are polysaccharides. Each fiber has a different structure and most contain monosaccharides, but they differ in the types they contain and in the bonds that link the monosaccharides to each other. These differences produce diverse health effects in the body. Fibers also differ from starches in that the bonds between their monosaccharides cannot be broken down by digestive enzymes. As a result, fibers do not supply monosaccharides to the body. The bacteria in the GI tract can break down some fibers, which is important to digestion and to overall health. The fibers that make up the plant foods are nonstarch polysaccharides that are not digested by the body's digestive enzymes, but some are digested by the GI tract bacteria. Fibers include cellulose, hemicelluloses, pectins, gums, and mucilages. The non-polysaccharides are lignins, cutins, and tannins.

Cellulose is the primary constituent of plant cell walls, and therefore occurs in all vegetables, fruits, and legumes. Like starch, the chains do not branch, and the bonds linking the glucose molecules together resist digestion by digestive enzymes.

Hemicelluloses are the main constituent of cereal fibers, and are composed of various monosaccharide backbones with branching side chains of monosaccharides. The side chains make the hemicelluloses a diverse group; some are soluble and others are insoluble.

Pectins consist of a backbone derived from carbohydrates with side chains of various monosaccharides. Commonly found in vegetables and fruits (especially apples and citrus fruits), pectins may be isolated and used by the food industry to thicken products such as jelly, keep salad dressing from separating, and control texture and consistency. Pectins are used for such products because they readily form gels in water.

Gums and mucilages are composed of various monosaccharides and their derivatives. Gums such as gum Arabic are used by the food industry as additives. Mucilages are similar to gums in structure; they include guar and carrageenan, which are added to foods as stabilizers.

Lignin is a non-polysaccharide fiber with a three-dimensional structure that gives it toughness. Because of this, few of the foods people eat contain much lignin. Lignin is found in the woody part of vegetables such as carrots and in the small seeds of fruit such as strawberries.

The above paragraphs classify fibers according to their chemical properties. However, they can also be classified as soluble fibers or insoluble fibers, depending on their solubility in water. Soluble fiber helps control blood sugar and may also lower cholesterol. Insoluble fiber doesn't appear to lower blood sugar or cholesterol, but fiber may help reduce the risk of colon cancer. It also helps maintain bowel function. The following lists show good sources of soluble and insoluble fiber.

Good sources of soluble fiber include:
- Oat bran (although many commercial oat bran muffins and waffles actually contain little fiber)
- Oatmeal
- Beans and legumes
- Peas
- Carrots
- Sweet potatoes
- Rice bran
- Barley
- Citrus fruits
- Strawberries
- Bananas

Good sources of insoluble fiber include:
- Whole wheat breads
- Wheat cereal
- Wheat bran

- Rice (except for white rice)
- Barley
- Cabbage
- Beets
- Brussels sprouts
- Turnips
- Cauliflower
- Fruits and vegetables with skin

Some classify fibers according to their physical properties that affect GI function and nutrient absorption. Physical properties of fiber include:

- Water-holding capacity—the capacity to capture water like a sponge, swelling and increasing the bulk of the intestines' contents
- Viscosity—the capacity to form viscous, gel-like solutions
- Cation-exchange capacity—the ability to bind minerals
- Bile-binding capacity—the ability to bind bile to acids
- Fermentability—the extent to which bacteria in the GI tract can break down fibers to fragments that the body is able to use

In summary, the complex carbohydrates are the polysaccharides (chains of monosaccharides), glycogen, starches, and fibers. Both glycogen and starch are storage forms of glucose in the body. Fibers also contain glucose (and other monosaccharides), but their bonds cannot be broken by digestive enzymes in the body, so they yield little energy, if any. The following summarizes the carbohydrate compounds:

Simple Carbohydrates (Sugars)
- Monosaccharides
- Galactose
- Glucose
- Fructose
- Disaccharides
- Maltose

- Sucrose
- Lactose

Complex Carbohydrates
- Polysaccharides
- Glycogen
- Starches
- Fibers (nonstarch polysaccharides)
- Soluble Fiber
- Insoluble Fiber

Digestion and Absorption of Carbohydrates

During the digestion and absorption of sugars and starches, they dismantle into small molecules—chiefly glucose—that the body is able to absorb and use. The large starch molecules require extensive breakdown. The disaccharides only need to be broken down once. The initial splitting begins in the mouth, the final splitting and absorption occur in the small intestine, and conversion to energy (glucose) takes place in the liver.

Digestion and Absorption Starts in the Mouth

In the mouth, vigorous chewing of high-fiber foods slows eating and stimulates the flow of saliva. The salivary enzyme amylase—an enzyme that breaks down carbohydrates—starts to work, breaking down starch to shorter polysaccharides and to maltose. Since food is in the mouth for only a short time, very little digestion takes place there.

The Stomach

Once the chewed food is swallowed, it mixes with the stomach's acid and protein-digesting enzymes, which deactivate the salivary amylase and make it unable to complete its job of starch digestion. To a small extent, the stomach's acid continues to break down the starch, but its juices contain no enzymes to digest carbohydrate. Fiber lingers in the stomach and delays gastric emptying, thereby providing a feeling of fullness and satiety.

The Small Intestine

The small intestine carries out most of the work of carbohydrate digestion. A major contributing carbohydrate-digesting enzyme is pancreatic amylase, which enters the intestine via the pancreatic duct and continues breaking down the polysaccharides to shorter glucose chains and disaccharides. The final phase takes place on the outer membranes of the intestinal cells.

The specific enzymes that dismantle three specific disaccharides are as follows:

- **Maltase**—breaks down maltose
- **Sucrase**—breaks down sucrose
- **Lactase**—breaks down lactose

The Large Intestine

Within two to four hours after a meal is consumed, all the sugars and most of the starches have been digested. Only a small fraction of the starches, and the indigestible fibers, remain in the digestive tract.

Starch may resist digestion, and the small amount that escapes digestion and absorption in the small intestine is known as resistant starch. Resistant starches are in whole legumes, raw potatoes, and unripe bananas. Since resistant starches remain in the large intestine, they promote bowel movements as fibers do. But unlike fibers, they do not lower blood cholesterol. Fibers in the large intestine attract water, which softens the stool for passage without straining. Bacteria in the GI tract ferment both resistant starches and fibers. The resistant starches and fibers contribute some energy, depending on the extent to which they are broken down and absorbed.

Absorption Into the Bloodstream

Glucose is unique in that it can be absorbed to some extent through the lining of the mouth, but for the most part, nutrient absorption takes place in the small intestine. Glucose and galactose traverse the intestinal cells lining in the small intestine by active transport; fructose is absorbed by facilitated diffusion, which slows its entry and produces a smaller rise in blood glucose. In the same way, unbranched chains of starch are digested slowly and produce a smaller rise in blood glucose than branched chains, which have many more places for enzymes to attack and release glucose rapidly.

As blood from the intestines circulates through the liver, cells take up fructose and galactose in order to convert them to other compounds, most often to glucose.

In summary, the digestion and absorption of carbohydrates in the body is the breaking down of starches into disaccharides and disaccharides into monosaccharides. Most of the monosaccharides are converted to glucose, to provide energy for the cells' work. The fibers help to regulate the passage of food through the GI system and slow the absorption of glucose, but they contribute little energy.

Glucose in the Body

The primary role of carbohydrates in the body is to supply the cells with glucose to deliver the indispensable product, energy. Starch contributes mostly to the body's glucose supply, as explained earlier; any of the monosaccharides can provide glucose as well.

The following sections will provide an overview of the pathways glucose can follow in the body and the ways which body regulates those pathways.

Storing Glucose as Glycogen

The liver stores one-third of the body's total glycogen and releases glucose as needed. During times of plenty, blood glucose rises, and liver cells link the excess glucose molecules into long branching chains of glycogen. When the blood glucose falls, the liver cells dismantle the glycogen into single molecules of glucose and release them into the bloodstream. Therefore, glucose becomes available to supply energy to the central nervous system and other organs, regardless of whether you have eaten recently. Muscle cells can also store glucose as glycogen (the other two-thirds), but they hoard most of their own supply, using it for energy only during exercise and other physically demanding activities.

Using Glucose for Energy

Glucose fuels the work of most of the cells in the body. Inside a cell, enzymes break glucose in half. These halves can be put back together to make glucose, or they can be further broken down into smaller fragments. The smaller fragments can yield energy when broken down completely to carbon dioxide and water, or they can be reassembled, but only into units of body fat.

As mentioned, glycogen stores last only for a few hours—not

for days, as you might think. To continue to provide glucose to meet the body's energy needs, you have to consume dietary carbohydrates frequently. Some people do not faithfully provide carbohydrates for their body's survival needs. How does the body manage without glucose from dietary carbohydrates? Does it draw energy from the other two energy-yielding nutrients, proteins and fats? Yes, it does draw energy from these two sources, but the process is not as simple as you might imagine.

Making Glucose from Protein

It must be noted that only glucose can provide energy for brain cells, other nerve cells, and developing red blood cells. Body protein can be converted to glucose to some extent, but protein has a job of its own that no other nutrient can do. Contrary to popular belief, body fat cannot be converted to glucose to any significant extent. When you do not replenish depleted glycogen stores by eating carbohydrate, proteins are dismantled to make glucose to fuel these special cells.

The conversion of protein to glucose is known as gluconeogenesis—literally, the making of new glucose. Only adequate dietary carbohydrate can prevent this use of protein for energy. This role of carbohydrate is known as protein-sparing action—the action of carbohydrate (and fat) in providing energy that allows protein to be used for other purposes.

Ketone Bodies from Fat Fragments

With less carbohydrate available for energy, more fat may be broken down, but not broken down all the way to energy. Instead, the fat fragments combine with each other, forming what is known as ketone bodies—the product of incomplete breakdown of fat when glucose is not available in the cells. Muscle and other tissues are able to use ketone bodies for energy. However, when their production exceeds their use, they accumulate in the blood, causing what is known as ketosis—an undesired high concentration of ketone bodies in the blood and urine.

In order to spare body protein and prevent ketosis, the average body needs around 50 to 100 grams of carbohydrates a day at the bare minimum. It is ideal to get around 275 to 500 grams of carbohydrate a day, depending on your body's needs.

Converting Glucose to Fat

When the body is given more carbohydrates than needed to meet its energy needs and fill its glycogen stores to capacity, the body must find a way to store any extra glucose. The liver breaks the glucose into smaller molecules and puts them together into the more permanent energy-storage compound—fat. The fat then travels to the fatty tissues of the body for storage. Fat cells are able to store unlimited quantities of fat, unlike the liver cells, which can store only about half a day's worth of glycogen.

Excess carbohydrates can be converted to fat and stored, but this is a relatively minor pathway because storing carbohydrates as body fat is expensive energy-wise. Simply put, the body uses more energy to convert dietary carbohydrate to body fat than it does to convert dietary fat to body fat. A balanced diet containing complex carbohydrates actually helps to control body weight. Most foods rich in starch and fibers are naturally low in fat, and when large amounts are eaten, they tend to crowd fat out in the diet.

Constancy of Blood Glucose

Every body cell depends on glucose for its fuel to some degree, and the cells of the brain and the rest of the nervous system depend primarily on glucose for their energy. The activity of these cells never ceases, and they do not have the ability to store glucose. They are continually drawing on the supply of glucose in the fluid surrounding them. In order to maintain the supply, a steady stream of blood moves past these cells, bringing more glucose from either the intestines (food) or the liver (from glycogen breakdown or glucose synthesis).

Glucose Homeostasis

In order for the body to function optimally, it must maintain blood glucose within limits that permit the cells to nourish themselves. If blood glucose falls below normal, you may become dizzy and weak; if it rises above normal, you may become fatigued. In any case, when left untreated high or low blood glucose levels can cause serious health problems.

Regulating Hormones

Blood glucose homeostasis is regulated primarily by two hormones:

- **Insulin**—A hormone secreted by special cells in the pancreas in response to increased blood glucose concentration. The primary role of insulin is to control the transport of glucose from the bloodstream into the muscle and fat cells.

- **Glucagon**—A hormone that is secreted by special cells in the pancreas in response to low blood glucose concentration. It elicits the release of glucose from storage.

After a meal, blood glucose slowly rises and special cells of the pancreas respond by secreting insulin into the bloodstream. As the circulating insulin contacts the receptors in the body's other cells, the receptors respond by escorting glucose from the bloodstream into the cells. Nearly all of the cells take only the glucose they can use for energy right away, but the liver and muscle cells are able to assemble the small glucose units into long branching chains of glycogen for storage. The liver cells are able to convert glucose to fat for export to other cells as well. The rise of blood glucose returns to normal as excess glucose is stored as glycogen (which can be converted back to glucose) and fat (which cannot be converted back to glucose).

Between meals, blood glucose falls, and other special cells of the pancreas respond by secreting glucagon into the blood. Glucagon raises blood glucose by signaling the liver to dismantle its glycogen stores and release glucose into the bloodstream, for use by all the other body cells.

An additional hormone that requires glucose from the liver cells is the "fight-or-flight" hormone epinephrine—a hormone of the adrenal glad that modulates the stress response. When you experience stress, epinephrine acts quickly, ensuring that all the body cells have energy fuel for emergencies. Similar to glucagon, epinephrine works to release glucose from liver glycogen to the bloodstream.

Balancing Blood Glucose

Maintaining a normal blood glucose level depends on two processes. Once blood glucose falls too low, food can replenish it; or, in the absence of food, glucagon can signal the liver to break down glycogen stores. When blood glucose rises too high, insulin can signal the cells to take in glucose for energy. It is important to eat balanced meals in order to maintain a steady level of blood glucose. Balanced meals that provide complex carbohydrates—including fibers, some proteins, and a few fats—are very helpful in maintaining healthy blood glucose levels. The fibers and fats slow down the digestion and absorption of carbohydrates, which allows glucose to enter the bloodstream gradually, providing a steady ongoing supply. Proteins elicit the secretion of glucose within the digestion process which helps to maintain blood glucose within a healthy level.

In summary, carbohydrates provide glucose that can be used by the cells for energy, stored by the liver and muscles as glycogen, or converted into fat if intake exceeds need. All of the body's cells depend on glucose; without glucose, the body is forced to break down its protein tissues to make glucose and to alter energy metabolism in order to make ketone bodies from fats. Blood glucose regulation depends chiefly on two pancreatic hormones: insulin to remove glucose from the bloodstream into the cells when levels are high, and glucagon to free glucose from glycogen stores and release it into the blood when levels are low.

Health Effects and Intake of Sugars

Honey and dates have long been enjoyed as sources of sweetness, and is a natural sugar, that should be consumed in small amounts in a healthy and balanced diet. The natural sugars of milk, fruits, vegetables, and grains account for about half of sugar intake. The other half consists of sugars that have been refined and added to foods for a variety of purposes. As an additive, sugar:

- Enhances flavor
- Supplies texture and color to baked goods
- Provides fuel for fermentation, causing bread to rise or producing alcohol
- Is a bulking agent in ice cream and baked goods
- Is a preservative in jams
- Balances the acidity of tomato and vinegar based products

The many sugars which do not occur naturally in foods are as follows:

- **Brown Sugar**—Refined white sugar crystals to which molasses has been added for natural flavor and color
- **Confectioners' Sugar**—Finely powdered sucrose
- **Corn Sweeteners**—Corn syrup and sugars derived from corn

- **Corn Syrup**—A syrup made from cornstarch that has been treated with acid, high temperatures, and enzymes
- **Dextrose**—Another name for glucose
- **Granulated Sugar**—Crystalline sucrose
- **High Fructose Corn Syrup**—Corn syrup that has been treated with enzymes that change glucose to fructose; man-made especially for use in processed foods and beverages
- **Honey**—Sugar (mostly sucrose) formed from nectar gathered by bees; the composition and flavor of honey varies, but it will always contain a mixture of sucrose, fructose and glucose
- **Levulose**—Another name for fructose
- **Maple Sugar**—A sugar (mostly sucrose) purified from the concentrated sap of sugar maple trees
- **Molasses**—A thick brown syrup produced during sugar refining which holds residual sugar and a few minerals; blackstrap molasses contains significant amounts of calcium and iron (the iron is from the machinery used to process the sugar)
- **Raw Sugar**—The first crop of crystals harvested during sugar processing; not sold in the United States because it contains dirt, insect fragments, and the like domestically sold "raw sugar" has gone through over half of the refining process
- **Turbinado Sugar**—Sugar produced using the same refining process as white sugar, but without the bleaching and anti-caking treatment; a trace of molasses give it a light brown color
- **White Sugar**—Pure sucrose known as table sugar, produced by dissolving, concentrating, and re-crystallizing raw sugar

The use of sweeteners in food manufacturing has greatly increased during the past several decades. The estimates of sugar consumption typically include all sweeteners used in the marketing system, including sugar lost or wasted.

In moderation, sugars add pleasure to meals without harming health, but an excess of sugar can be detrimental. Consuming a high sugar intake falls below the recommendations for a healthful diet.

Nutrient Deficiencies

Empty-calorie foods that contain lots of added sugar—such as cakes, candies, and sodas—deliver glucose and energy, but few other nutrients, if any. In comparison, foods such as whole grains, vegetables, legumes, and fruits contain some natural sugars, starches and fibers, which help deliver glucose and energy to the body, along with protein, vitamins, and minerals.

Sugar can contribute to nutrient deficiencies only by displacing nutrients. For the sake of nutrition, the appropriate outlook to take is not that sugar is "bad" and must be avoided, but that in a healthful diet nutritious foods come first. If the nutritious foods end up crowding sugar out of the diet, that is fine—but not the other way around. It is important to have balance, variety, and moderation in a healthful diet.

In summary, excessive sugar intake may displace needed nutrients and fiber which the body needs; too many sugars may lead to obesity as well. When limiting sugar intake, it must be recognized that not all sugars are created equal. Concentrated sugars in sweets are relatively empty calories, but the natural sugars in fruits, vegetables and milk are not.

Health Effects of Starches and Fibers

In addition to starch, fibers, and natural sugars, whole grains, vegetables, legumes, and fruits supply the body with valuable vitamins and minerals. The following points describe some of the health benefits of a diet that includes a variety of these foods on a daily basis:

- **Cancer**—A high-carbohydrate diet, with plenty of green and yellow vegetables and citrus fruits, protects against some types of cancer. It is unclear whether the protection is derived from the fiber, vitamins, or phytochemicals in these foods. Fibers are known to prevent colon cancer by diluting, binding, and rapidly removing potential cancer-causing agents from the colon.

- **Diabetes**—A moderate carbohydrate diet often helps lower the chances of diabetes, most likely because such a diet is low in fat. Consuming a moderate carbohydrate and low-fat diet seems to be effective in preventing the most common type of diabetes—type II diabetes. High fiber foods play an important role in reducing the risk of diabetes. When soluble fibers trap nutrients and delay their transit through the GI tract, glucose absorption is slowed, which helps to prevent the glucose surge and rebound that is associated with the onset of diabetes.

- **Excessive Fiber Intake**—Regardless of fiber's benefits to overall health, a diet too high in it has a few drawbacks. When adhering to a mostly high-fiber diet, it might be hard to take in enough nutrients and food energy. The malnourished, elderly, children, and vegans are especially vulnerable to this kind of problem. Launching into a high-fiber diet can cause bouts of abdominal discomfort, gas, diarrhea, and, more seriously, can obstruct the GI tract. To avoid such complications, follow these three tips: (1) Increase fiber intake gradually over several weeks to allow the GI tract time to adapt. (2) Drink plenty of fluids to soften the fiber as it moves through the GI tract. (3) Select a variety of fiber-rich foods. Fiber is like all nutrients, in that more is only better up to a certain point.

- **GI Health**—Dietary fibers enhance the health of the large intestine, and the healthier the intestinal walls are, the better they are able to block absorption of unwanted elements. Consuming insoluble fibers such as cellulose will enlarge the stools, easing passage, and speeding up transit time. Plus, the undigested fibers, together with the microbial growth, help to alleviate and/or prevent constipation. Fibers help in preventing several GI problems and related disorders, such as hemorrhoids, appendicitis, and diverticula.

- **Heart Disease**—A high-carbohydrate diet rich in whole grains seems to protect against heart disease and stroke. Such diets are lower in animal fat and cholesterol, and high in soluble fibers, vegetables, fruits, and nuts—all factors linked with a lower risk of heart disease. Foods rich in soluble fibers (barley, legumes, whole grains, and oat bran) lower blood cholesterol by binding with bile acids, which increase their excretion. The liver must then use its own cholesterol to make new bile acids. Also, the bacterial by-products of fiber digestion in the colon inhibit cholesterol synthesis in the liver, with the final result being lower blood cholesterol.

- **Weight Control**—A diet rich in complex carbohydrates and low in fat and sugar aids in weight loss and maintenance, as it offers less energy per bite, providing satiety, and delaying hunger. The high fiber content in the food not only adds bulk to the diet, but it is economical and nutritious as well. (**Side Note**: Read the labels on all baked goods and other prepackaged foods—many products include the word "healthy" in their labels have added sugars and contain hydrogenated fats.)

In summary, adequate fiber intake:

- Helps prevent colon cancer

- Helps prevent and control diabetes

- Helps prevent and alleviate hemorrhoids

- Helps prevent appendicitis

- Helps prevent diverticulosis

- Lowers blood cholesterol

- Promotes weight control

An excessive fiber intake:

- Changes the structure of nutrient dense foods

- Causes intestinal discomfort

- Interferes with mineral absorption

Intake of Starches and Fibers

Dietary recommendations advocate that carbohydrates provide more than half of a healthy diet (55-60 percent) to meet energy requirements. The best food choices are whole grains, legumes, vegetables, and fruits, which are also good sources of vitamins and minerals that the body needs. Fiber in selected foods is listed as follows:

Grain products provide about 1 to 2 grams of fiber per serving:

- 1 slice whole wheat, pumpernickel, or rye bread
- 1 oz. ready-to-eat cereal (**Side Note:** 100% bran cereal contains up to 10 grams or more)
- ½ cup cooked barley, bulgur, grits, or oatmeal

Vegetables provide about 2 to 3 grams of fiber per serving:

- 1 cup raw bean sprouts
- ½ cup chopped raw carrots or peppers
- ½ cup cooked broccoli, Brussels sprouts, cabbage, carrots, cauliflower, collards, green beans, eggplant, spinach, pumpkin, potatoes, green peas, sweet potatoes, winter squash, kale, mushrooms, okra, etc.

Fresh, frozen or dried fruits provide about 2 grams of fiber per serving:

- 1 medium apple, banana, kiwi, nectarine, orange, peach, or pear
- ½ cup applesauce, cherries, blackberries, blueberries, raspberries, or strawberries

Legumes provide about 5 to 8 grams of fiber per serving:

- ½ cup cooked baked beans, black beans, kidney beans, pinto beans, garbanzo beans, lentils, lima beans, or split peas

In summary, a diet rich in complex carbohydrates—starches and fibers—aids in preventing cancer, diabetes and GI disorders, and helps control body weight. It is recommended that you eat plenty of whole grains, legumes, vegetables, and fruits—enough to provide about 55-60 percent of the daily energy intake from carbohydrates. What carbohydrates do you included in your everyday diet?

CHAPTER 3
About Proteins

People associate protein with strength and meat with protein. As a result, they consume large amounts of meat protein to build their muscles, but their thinking is only partly correct. Protein is a vital structural and working substance in all cells, not just muscle cells. Meat is a good source of protein, but so are eggs, milk, legumes, and many whole grain and vegetables. Protein is important, but it is only one of the nutrients required to maintain a healthy body.

The Breakdown of Proteins

Proteins contain the same atoms as carbohydrates and fats—carbon, hydrogen, and oxygen—but proteins also contain nitrogen atoms. These nitrogen atoms give the name amino to the amino acids—the building blocks of proteins. Amino acids contain an amino group, an acid group, a hydrogen atom, and a distinctive side group, all attached to a central carbon atom.

All amino acids have the same basic makeup, but each has a unique side group. These side groups vary from one amino acid to the next, making proteins more complex than either carbohydrates or fats. A protein is made up of about 20 different amino acids, each with a different side group.

The simplest amino acid, glycine, has a hydrogen atom as its side group. A slightly more complex amino acid, alanine, has an extra carbon and includes three hydrogen atoms as well. Therefore, even though all amino acids share a common structure, they differ in size, shape, electrical charge, and other characteristics because of the differences in these side groups.

Nonessential and Essential Amino Acids

More than half of the amino acids are known as nonessential—amino acids which the body is able to synthesize for itself. Foods can deliver these amino acids, but it is not essential that they do, since the body is able to produce them itself. As long as the body has the nitrogen form of the amino group and fragments from carbohydrate and fat to form the rest of the structure, the body is able to make any nonessential amino acid.

The others are known as the essential amino acids—amino acids which the body is unable to synthesize in amounts needed to meet its requirements. These nine amino acids must be supplied by the diet.

Below is a list of the nonessential and essential amino acids:

Nonessential Amino Acids

- Alanine
- Arginine
- Asparagine
- Aspartic Acid
- Cysteine
- Glutamic Acid
- Glutamine
- Glycine
- Proline
- Serine
- Tyrosine

Essential Amino Acids

- Histidine
- Isoleucine
- Leucine
- Lysine
- Methionine
- Phenylalanine
- Threonine
- Tryptophan
- Valine

Protein cells link amino acids end-to-end in a virtually limitless variety of sequences to form countless different proteins. Each amino acid is connected to the other by what is known as a peptide bond—a bond that connects the acid end of one amino acid to another end of an amino acid, forming a protein chain.

Condensation reactions connect the amino acids, just as they do the monosaccharides to form disaccharides. When two amino acids bond together, they form what is known as a *dipeptide*—*di* meaning two and *peptide* meaning amino acid. A third amino acid can be added to the amino acid chain to form what is known as a *tripeptide*—*tri* meaning three. When more than three amino acids join the amino acid chain form, it is known as a *polypeptide*—when more than ten amino acids bond together.

Protein Functions

The unique shaping of proteins allows them to perform various tasks in the body. Some to form hollow balls that are able to carry and store materials within them, such as those of tendons, which are more than ten times as long as they are wide, and form strong, rod-like structures. It should be noted that some polypeptides are functioning proteins as they are; others need to combine with other polypeptides to form large working compounds. This means that some proteins require minerals to activate them. For example, one molecule of hemoglobin (the globular protein of the red blood cells that carries oxygen from the lungs to the cells throughout the body—hemo meaning blood and globin meaning globular protein) is made of four linked polypeptide chains, each containing the mineral iron.

Protein Denaturation

Whenever proteins are subjected to heat, acid, or other situations which disturb their stability, they undergo what is known as denaturation—the change in the protein's shape and loss of its function brought on by heat, acid, or other agents.

In summary, proteins are more complex than carbohydrates or fats. Each amino acid contains an amino acid group, a hydrogen atom, and a distinct side group. The distinctive sequence of amino acids in each protein determines its exclusive shape and function.

Digestion and Absorption of Proteins

When foods containing protein are consumed, enzymes break the long polypeptide strands into shorter strands; the shorter strands into tripeptides and dipeptides; and, finally, the tripeptides and dipeptides into amino acids. The proteins in the food do not become body proteins straight away. Instead, they supply the amino acids from which the body is able to make its own protein.

Digestion and Absorption Starts in the Mouth

Digestion begins in the mouth. The chewing and crushing of protein-rich foods moistens and mixes them with saliva to be swallowed.

The Stomach

Proteins, of course, are crushed and the process of digestion begins in the mouth, but the real feat begins in the stomach. In the stomach, the proteins become partial breakdown of proteins. The hydrochloric acid uncoils each protein's tangled strands so that the digestive enzymes can attack the peptide bonds. This is what is referred to as denaturation. Also, the hydrochloric acid is able to convert the inactive form of the enzyme pepsinogen to its active form, pepsin—a gastric enzyme that breaks down protein. It is activated by hydrochloric acid in the stomach. Pepsin is known to chop proteins—large polypeptides—into smaller polypeptides and some amino acids.

The Small Intestine

As polypeptides enter the small intestine, numerous pancreatic and intestinal proteases—enzymes that break down protein—break them down further into short peptide chains, tripeptides, dipeptides, and amino acids. After that, peptidase—a digestive enzyme on the membrane surfaces of the intestinal cells—breaks down peptide bonds. This splits the majority of the dipeptides and tripeptides into single amino acids.

Absorption into the Bloodstream

A number of particular carriers transport amino acids, along with a few dipeptides and tripeptides, into the intestinal cells. From there, the intestinal cells and amino acids may be used for energy or to produce needed compounds. The ones that are not used by the intestinal cells are transported across the cell membrane into the surrounding fluid, where they go into the capillaries on their way to the liver. (**Side Note**: Many people fail to realize that most proteins are broken down into amino acids before absorption. They believe that they must consume "enzyme A" because it will aid in digesting their food, or they do not eat "food B" because it contains "enzyme C," which will digest cells in the body. In actuality, enzymes in foods are digested, just as all proteins are. Even the digestive enzymes, which work best at their precise pH, are denatured and digested when the pH of their environment changes. Another misconception is that consuming predigested proteins—protein supplements—saves the body from having to digest proteins and keeps the digestive system from being overtaxed. This kind of belief underestimates the body's abilities. In reality, the digestive system handles whole undigested proteins better than predigested ones, because it disassembles and absorbs the amino acids at rates that are most advantageous for the body's use.)

In summary, digestion is facilitated mostly by the stomach's acid and enzymes, which first denatures dietary proteins, and then chops them into smaller polypeptides and some amino acids. After that, the pancreatic and intestinal enzymes split these polypeptides further, into oligopeptides, tripeptides, and dipeptides; and then split most of these into single amino acids. Once this has taken place, carriers in the membranes of the intestinal cells transport the amino acids into cells, where they are released into the bloodstream.

Proteins in the Body

The body contains about 10,000 to 50,000 different kinds of proteins. Of these proteins, about 100 have been studied. Each and every body has minute differences—that is determined by genes—which are shown in the slight changes by the amino acid sequences of proteins.

The following is a brief summary of the way cells synthesize proteins:

- **Transporting the information**—Deoxyribonucleic acid, or DNA, is the double-stranded (shaped like a double helix) chemical manual for a living organism. Every organism has DNA, which shows it how to grow, what characteristics to develop, and when to die. DNA is found in every cell of an organism's body. Ribonucleic acid, or RNA, is single-stranded. It carries single pages of instructions out of the nucleus to places throughout the cell where they are needed. It copies ten times faster than DNA, and its performance is error-free. It helps translate the mRNA in the ribosome into amino acids. RNA has three functions: (1) it serves as the messenger that tells the ribosome in the cell what protein to make; (2) it serves as part of the structure of the ribosome; and (3) it functions to bring amino acids to the ribosome when a specific amino acid is called for. To notify a cell of the sequence of amino acids for a needed protein, an elongated DNA strand serves as a template for making a strand of RNA, which carries a code. The messenger RNA presents its list, specifying the sequence in which the amino acids are to line up in order to make a strand of protein.

- **Arranging the amino acids**—Another form of RNA, called transfer RNA, collects amino acids from fluid and brings them into the messenger RNA. Each of the 20 amino acids has a specific transfer RNA. When the messenger needs a specific amino acid, the transfer RNA carries that particular amino acid into its position. This process continues until the sequence needed is complete and the enzymes have bound them together. Finally, the completed protein strand is released, the messenger is degraded, and the transfer RNA is released to return for more loads of amino acids.

- **Sequence Errors**—The sequence of amino acids in each and every protein determines its shape, which in turn supports a specific function. When a genetic error occurs, it changes the amino acid sequence of the protein. If a mistake has been made in copying the sequence, an altered protein will result. An example of such a genetic variation is sickle-cell anemia. In the case of sickle-cell anemia, a defect in the hemoglobin molecule (the globular protein of the red blood cells that carry oxygen from the lungs to the cells throughout the body) changes the shape of the red blood cells. Therefore, sickle-cell anemia interferes with the oxygen transport and blood flow.

- **Nutrients and gene expressed**—Whenever a cell makes a protein, it is known as "expressed." Cells are able to regulate gene expression in order to make the type of protein in the amounts and at the rate needed. Virtually all of the body's cells have the ability to make all human proteins from genes, but each type of cell makes only the proteins it needs. For example, the cells of the pancreas do not make the protein hemoglobin, which is needed only by the red blood cells. Pancreas cells only express the gene for insulin; in other cells, this gene is idle.

In summary, cells produce proteins according to the genetic information provided by the DNA in the nucleus of each cell. This information is responsible for the order in which the amino acids must be linked together to form its given protein. At times, sequencing errors occur, and health problems arise as a result.

Roles of Protein

As the body is growing, repairing, or replacing tissue, proteins are involved. At times, their responsibility is to facilitate or regulate; at other times, they are to become part of a structure. Proteins are one of the most versatile nutrients. The following lists the many roles of protein.

- **Building Materials**—From the moment of conception, proteins are involved. They form the building blocks of most of the body's structures. For example, in order to build bone or a tooth, cells first lay down what is known as matrix (the basic substance that gives form to a developing structure in the body) of protein collagen (the protein from which connective tissues such as tendons, ligaments, scars, and the foundations of bones and teeth are made) and then fill it with crystals of calcium, phosphorus, magnesium, fluoride, and other minerals. Proteins are also needed for replacement or repair. Cells in the body break down proteins to go into hair and fingernails. Cells of the

GI tract are replaced about every three days. Both inside and outside, the body continuously deposits protein into new cells that replace those that have been lost or need to be repaired.

- **Enzymes**—Enzymes not only break down substances, they also build substances and transform one substance into another. Enzymes are comparable to the clergy and judges who make and dissolve marriages. When a minister marries two separate individuals, they become one, with a new bond between them. They are seen as being joined together, but the minister that performed the ceremony remains unchanged. The minister represents an enzyme that breaks down large compounds into complete, but smaller compounds, without being changed. A single minister can perform countless marriage ceremonies, just as one enzyme can perform scores of synthetic responses. Similarly, a judge who allows married couples to separate may decree numerous divorces before retiring or dying. The judge represents enzymes that break down larger compounds to smaller ones. The point is that, like the minister and the judge, enzymes themselves are not altered by the reactions they facilitate. They are catalysts, permitting reactions to occur more quickly and efficiently, without being changed by what is taking place around them.

- **Hormones**—The body's various hormones are messenger molecules, and some hormones are proteins. A variety of glands in the body release hormones in response to changes in the internal environment. The blood carries the hormones from these glands to their target tissues, where they elicit the appropriate responses to restore or maintain normal conditions. For example, when blood glucose rises, the pancreas releases its insulin. The insulin then stimulates the transport proteins of the muscles and fat tissue to pump glucose into the cells faster than it can escape. As blood glucose falls, the pancreas reduces its insulin output. There are many other proteins which act as hormones, regulating a variety of actions in the body. They are as follows:

Hormones and Their Actions

- Growth hormone—actively promotes growth
- Insulin and glucagon—actives and regulates blood glucose
- Thyroxin—actives and regulates the body's metabolic rate
- Calcitonin and parathormone—actives and regulates blood calcium
- Antidiuretic hormone—actives and regulates fluid and electrolyte balance

Hormones are chemical messengers that are secreted by endocrine glands in response to altered conditions in the body. Each travels to one or more specific target tissues or organs, where it elicits a specific response. The following are just a few of the functions in which proteins and hormones work to keep the body functioning properly.

- **Regulator of fluid balance**—Proteins help to maintain the body's fluid balance. The body's fluids are contained within the cells (intercellular) or outside of the cells (extracellular). Fluid balance means that the various body compartments contain the required amount of water, proportioned according to their needs. The exchange of materials between the blood and the cells takes place across the capillary walls, which allow the passage of fluids and a variety of materials—but not usually plasma proteins. Still, proteins escape out of the capillaries into the interstitial fluid between the cells. These proteins cannot be reabsorbed back into the plasma; they generally reenter circulation via the lymph system. If plasma proteins enter the interstitial spaces faster than they are able to be cleared, fluid accumulates (because proteins attract water) and swelling occurs. The swelling due to an excess of interstitial fluid is known as edema—the swelling of body tissue cased by excessive amounts of fluid in the interstitial spaces. This is seen in protein deficiency, among other health conditions.

- **Acid and base regulator**—Proteins help to maintain the balance between acids (compounds that release hydrogen ions in a solution) and bases (compounds that accept hydrogen ions in a solution) within the body fluids. Normal body processes continually produce acids and bases, which the blood carries to the kidneys and lungs for excretion. Acid solutions contain hydrogen ions; the more hydrogen ions, the more concentrated the acid. Proteins have a negative charge on their surfaces, which tend to attract hydrogen ions, which have a positive charge. By accepting hydrogen ions, proteins maintain the acid-base balance of the blood and body fluids.

- **Transporters**—A number of proteins move about in the body fluids, carrying nutrients and other molecules. The protein hemoglobin carries oxygen from the lungs to the cells; the lipoproteins carry fats around the body; and special transport proteins carry vitamins and minerals.

- **Antibodies**—Proteins also defend the body against disease. A virus—whether it is one that causes flu, chickenpox, measles, or the common cold—enters the cells and multiplies there. A virus is known to produce 100 replicas of itself within an hour or so. Each replica can burst out and invade 100 different cells. Left free to do their worst, they will soon overwhelm the body with disease. Antigens are substances that elicit the formation of antibodies or an inflammation reaction from the immune system. A virus, toxins, and proteins in foods that cause allergens are all examples of antigens. Antibodies are giant protein molecules produced by the immune system in response to the invasion of foreign molecules in the body. Antibodies protect the body by combining with and inactivating the foreign invaders. Fortunately, when the body senses invading antigens, it manufactures antibodies designed specifically to combat them. The antibodies work so efficiently that in normal, healthy individuals, most diseases never have a chance to get started. However, without sufficient protein, the body cannot maintain the antibodies needed to resist infectious diseases. Plus, each antibody is designed to destroy just one antigen. Once the body has manufactured antibodies against a particular antigen, it remembers how to make them. Consequently, the next time the body encounters that same antigen, it will quickly produce more antibodies. The body develops a molecular memory known as immunity—the body's ability to recognize and eliminate foreign invaders.

- **Source of energy and glucose**—Without energy, cells die; without glucose, the brain and nervous system falters. So even though proteins are needed to do the work that only they can execute, they are able to provide energy and glucose, if needed.

- **Miscellaneous roles**—Protein is an integral part of most body structures such as skin, muscles, and bones. It also participates in some of the body's most amazing activities, such as blood clotting and vision. When a tissue is injured, a rapid chain of event leads to the production of fibrin—a stringy insoluble mass of protein fibers that is able to form a clot from liquid blood. The protein collagen forms a scar to replace the clot and permanently heal the damaged tissue.

In summary, protein functions are as follows:

Growth and maintenance—Proteins form the primary parts of most body structures such as skin, tendons, membranes, muscles, organs, and bones, and support the growth and repair of body tissues.

Enzymes—Proteins assist in chemical reactions.

Hormones—Proteins regulate body processes. (**Side Note**: Not all hormones are made of protein.)

Fluid balance—Proteins help to maintain volume and composition of body fluids.

Acid and base balance—Proteins help maintain the acid and base balance of the body fluids by acting as buffers.

Transportation—Proteins transport substances such as fat, vitamins, minerals, and oxygen throughout the body.

Antibodies—Proteins inactivate foreign invaders and, as a result, protect the body against diseases.

Energy—Proteins are able to provide fuel for the body's energy needs.

Protein and Metabolism
The Amino Acid Pool

Inside each cell, proteins are regularly being made and broken down, a process known as protein turnover. When proteins break down, they allow amino acids to join the general circulation of the bloodstream. These amino acids then mix with amino acids from dietary protein to form what is known as an amino acid pool. This is the supply of amino acids, derived from either food proteins or body proteins, which collect in the cells and circulating blood, and stand ready to be incorporated in proteins and other compounds or to be used for energy.

Nitrogen Balance

The rate of protein breakdown and the amount of protein intake may vary, but the pattern of amino acids inside the pool remains fairly constant. Whatever their source, all of these amino acids can be used to make body proteins or nitrogen-containing compounds, or they can be stripped of their nitrogen and used for energy.

Nitrogen and protein turnover go hand in hand. In most healthy individuals, protein synthesis balances with the breakdown. Protein intake from food balances with nitrogen excretion in the urine, feces, and sweat. When nitrogen intake equals nitrogen output, the individual is in nitrogen equilibrium or balance.

If the body synthesizes more than it breaks down and adds protein, the nitrogen standing becomes positive. The nitrogen standing is positive in growing infants and children, pregnant women, and people recovering from protein deficiency or illness. In each, the nitrogen intake exceeds the nitrogen output, and the body retains protein in new tissues as it adds blood, bone, skin, and muscle cells.

If the body breaks down more than it synthesizes and loses protein, the nitrogen standing becomes negative. The nitrogen standing is negative in those who are starving or suffering other severe stress, such as individuals who have burns, injuries, infections, and fever. In each, the nitrogen output exceeds the nitrogen intake, and the body loses nitrogen as it breaks down muscle and other body proteins for energy.

Using Amino Acids to Make Proteins, Nonessential Amino Acids, and Other Compounds

As stated earlier, cells have the ability to assemble amino acids into proteins they need in order to do their work. For example, if a particular nonessential amino acid is not readily available, cells are able to make it from other amino acids. If an essential amino acid is missing, the body is able to break down some of its own proteins to obtain it. Also, cells are able to use amino acids to make other compounds. For example, the amino acid tyrosine is used to make the neurotransmitter (chemicals that are released at the end of a nerve cell when a nerve impulse is received; they diffuse across the gap to the next cell and alter the membrane of that second cell to either inhibit or excite it) norepinephrine, which relays nervous system messages throughout the body. Tyrosine also can be made into the pigment melanin, which is responsible for brown hair, eye, and skin color; or tyrosine can be converted into the hormone thyroxin, which helps to regulate the metabolic rate.

Using Amino Acids for Energy

When glucose or fats are limited, cells are forced to use amino acids for energy and glucose. The body does not have a specialized storage form of protein as it does for carbohydrates and fats. Glucose is stored as glycogen in the liver and fat as triglycerides in adipose tissue, but protein is available only as the body breaks down its tissue proteins and uses them for energy. Over time, energy starvation always incurs wasting of lean body tissue (muscle), as well as fat loss. Having an adequate supply of carbohydrates and fats spares amino acids from being used for energy and allows protein to be used in the body as it was designed to be used.

Using Amino Acids to Make Fat

If an individual consumes more protein than the body needs, the amino acids are deaminated, meaning that the nitrogen is excreted, and the remaining carbon fragments are converted to fat and stored for later use.

Deaminating Amino Acids

When amino acids are broken down, which is what occurs when they are used for energy, they are first deaminated—stripped of their nitrogen-containing amino acid groups. Deamination is a process that produces ammonia, released by cells into the bloodstream. Next, the liver picks up the ammonia, converts it into urea (a less toxic compound), and returns the urea to the bloodstream. Finally, the kidneys filter urea out of the blood, where the nitrogen from amino acids ends up in the urine. The remaining carbon fragments may enter a number of metabolic pathways, such as being used to make fat.

In summary, proteins are constantly being synthesized and broken down as needed by the body. The body's alteration of amino acids into proteins, by releasing the amino acids via protein degradation and excretion, can be tracked by measuring the nitrogen balance in the body, which will be positive during growth stages and in healthy individuals. Energy deficit or an inadequate protein intake may force the body to use amino acids as energy, creating a negative nitrogen balance. When protein is consumed in excess of need, it is degraded and stored as body fat.

Proteins in Foods

Individuals in the United States and Canada eat protein in such large quantities that they receive, for the most part, all the amino acids their bodies need. But in countries where food is scarce, and individuals eat only marginal amounts of protein-rich foods, the quality of the protein becomes crucial. It determines how well children grow and how well individuals maintain their health.

The protein quality of the diet is of great concern when making nutrition recommendations, especially in countries where malnutrition is widespread. Low-quality proteins seem to fail to provide enough of all the essential amino acids required to support the body's needs.

The following are five points to keep in mind about the quality of protein:

- **Limiting Amino Acids**—In order to make proteins, a cell needs to have all the needed amino acids available simultaneously. The liver is able to produce any nonessential amino acid that may be in short supply, so that the cells are able to continue linking amino acids to protein strands. However, if an essential amino acid is missing, a cell must break down its own proteins in order to obtain it. To keep protein breakdown from happening, dietary protein needs to supply at least the nine essential amino acids, as well as enough nitrogen-containing amino acid groups and energy for synthesis of the others. If the diet contains too few of any essential amino acids, protein synthesis will be limited. The body is able to make whole proteins, but if an amino acid is missing, the others are unable to form a half or whole protein. When essential amino acids are supplied in amounts less than the body needs to support protein synthesis, it is known as limiting amino acid—the essential amino acid found in the shortest supply relative to the amounts needed for protein synthesis in the body. There are four amino acids that are most likely to be limiting: lysine, methionine, threonine, and tryptophan.

- **Complete Protein**—As stated early on, a complete protein contains all the essential amino acids in the relative amounts which the body requires, but it may or may not contain all the nonessential amino acids. Generally, proteins derived from animal sources are complete proteins, but in comparison to plant protein sources, which have a more diverse amino acid pattern, they tend to be limited in one or more essential amino acids.

- **Complementary Proteins**—Plant proteins are of lower quality then animal proteins. Also, plant proteins offer less protein per weight or measure of food. Many vegetarians improve the quality of proteins in their diets by combining plant-protein foods that have different but complementary amino acid patterns. This approach is known as mutual supplementation— the combining of two protein foods in a meal so that each food provides the essential amino acid(s) lacking in the other. Doing so yields complementary proteins that contain all the essential amino acids in quantities that are sufficient to support health.

- **Digestibility**—Complete proteins are digestible enough to provide the amino acids needed for protein synthesis. Such proteins are considered high-quality proteins—easy digestibility. The protein digestibility depends on such factors as a food protein's source and the other foods eaten with it. The digestibility of most animal proteins is high. Plant proteins are less digestible, due to the fact that they are inside the plant cell walls, which resist digestion.

- **Reference Protein**—The most complete and digestible protein is egg protein. Egg protein can be used as a standard for measuring protein quality. It is assigned a value of 100, and the quality of other protein-rich foods is determined based on how they compare with the egg. This standard is known as reference protein—a standard against which to measure the quality of other proteins.

In summary, a diet that is inadequate in any of the essential amino acids limits protein synthesis. The best assurance of amino acid sufficiency is to eat foods containing complete proteins or mixtures of foods containing incomplete, but complementary proteins, which can supply the missing amino acids.

Measures of Protein Quality

Scientists and researchers have developed several methods for evaluating the quality of food proteins and identifying high-quality proteins. The following are brief descriptions of these measures:

- **Amino Acid Scoring**—This is a method of evaluating protein quality by comparing a protein's amino acid pattern with that of a reference protein; sometimes referred to as chemical scoring.

- **Biological Value**—This is the amount of protein nitrogen that is retained from a given amount of protein nitrogen absorbed; in other words, it is a measure of protein quality.

- **Net Protein Utilization**—This is the amount of protein nitrogen that is retained from a given amount of protein nitrogen consumed; in other words, it is a measure of protein quality. Net Protein Utilization is much like Biological Value, but the difference is that Net Protein Utilization measures retention of food nitrogen consumed rather than food nitrogen absorbed as in Biological Value.

- **Protein Efficiency Ratio**—This is a measure of protein quality assessed by determining how well a given protein supports weight gain (in rats), and is used to establish the protein quality for infant formulas and baby foods.

- **PDCAAS (Protein Digestibility-Corrected Amino Acid Score)**—This is a measure of protein quality assessed by comparing the amino acid score of a food protein with the amino acid requirements of preschool-age children, and then correcting for the true digestibility of the protein.

In summary, the quality of protein is measured by its amino acid content, its digestibility, and its ability to support and maintain growth.

Health Effects of Protein

By now you know that protein is crucial to life. It should come as no surprise, then, that protein deficiency can have devastating effects on an individual's health. Nevertheless, like other nutrients, protein in excess is also harmful to the body. The following points describe the health problems that arise when the proper intake of protein is not kept in balance in the diet:

- **Protein-Energy Malnutrition (PEM)**—This is a deficiency of protein, energy, or both. Many adults suffer from this condition, but it most often strikes early in childhood.

- **Acute PEM**—This is a protein-energy malnutrition caused by recent severe food restriction.

- **Chronic PEM**—This is a protein-energy malnutrition caused by long-term food deprivation.

- **Marasmus**—This is a form of PEM that results from severe deprivation or impaired absorption of protein, energy, vitamins, and minerals.

- **Kwashiorkor**—This is a form of PEM that results from either inadequate protein consumption or, more commonly, infections.

- **Infections**—Malnourished individuals are much more vulnerable to infections. For example, an infection of the digestive tract causes diarrhea, further depleting the body of nutrients. If untreated, the combination of infection, fever, and fluid imbalances often leads to detrimental health problems, and in some cases can result in heart failure and death.

- **Adult Bone Loss**—Some research suggest that calcium loss occurs when a protein-rich diet is consumed, because such diets are lower in fruits and vegetables and produces a lot of acid. The body's skeleton responds to this abundance of acidity by giving up its calcium. Adding fruits and vegetables to a diet high in protein creates less acidity and decreases the loss of calcium from the bones.

- **Cancer**—The effects of protein-rich foods on cancers cannot be easily determined. Some studies suggest a correlation between protein-rich diets and some forms of cancer, especially colon, breast, kidney, pancreas, and prostate cancer.

- **Heart Disease**—Some protein-rich foods, such as animal protein, tend to be high in saturated fats, which contribute to heart disease. A low to moderate intake of such foods will help in the battle against heart disease.

- **Kidney Disease**—A protein-rich diet increases the work of the kidneys, so an intake of low to moderate protein will be of great benefit in keeping the kidneys healthy. Plus, the end products of protein metabolism depend on an adequate fluid intake, and ultimately on how healthy the kidneys are.

- **Weight Control**—Protein-rich foods are often high in fat, which can contribute to being overweight. The higher the individual's consumption of protein-rich foods such as meat and dairy products, the more likelihood that fruits, vegetables, and grains will be crowded out, making the diet inadequate and out of balance in other nutrients.

In summary, protein deficiencies arise from both energy and protein-poor diets, and can lead to devastating disease and other health problems. An excessive amount of protein in the diet offers no health advantages, and may cause more serious health problems. It is important to be aware of this, especially in this day and age, where protein-rich foods are readily available. If these health problems are caught in time and attended to, the individual's life may be spared. He or she may not experience too many health problems while on the road of recovery, and even later in life.

Intake of Quality Proteins

As established earlier, the body is always breaking down and losing its proteins and is unable to store amino acids, so protein must be replaced. The body needs dietary protein for two major reasons: (1) food protein is the only source of the essential amino acids, and (2) it is the only sensible source of nitrogen with which to build the nonessential amino acids and other nitrogen-containing compounds that the body needs.

Dietary recommendations advocate that proteins make up about 15 percent of the diet, in order to meet energy requirements. The best food choices are beef, poultry, lamb, fish, dairy products (including cottage cheese, cheese, yogurt and milk), eggs, egg whites or egg substitutes, dry beans, peas, oats, legumes, nuts, seeds, tofu, and some soy products.

In all cases, protein intake will depend on age, medical condition, activity level, and body size. For most adults, two to three servings of protein a day is adequate. Some common serving sizes of protein include:

- 3 to 4 ounces of cooked lean meat, poultry or fish
- 1/2 cup of cooked dry beans, lentils or legumes
- 1 egg or 2 tablespoons of peanut butter, which count as 1 ounce of lean meat

The recommended daily allowance (RDA) for healthy adults is 0.8 grams of protein per kilogram of body weight per day. The recommendation for healthy growing infants and children is higher. Nevertheless, when compared to total energy intake, the recommended daily allowance of protein for infants and children is comparable to that of a healthy adult. The recommended daily allowance generously covers what is needed for replacing worn-out tissue, building new tissue, and the increased intake for infants, children, and pregnant women. The recommendations for athletes are somewhat higher than those for a healthy adult. The following is an example of how to calculate the recommended protein intake for healthy individuals.

In order to find the protein RDA:

- Look up the healthy weight for a given individual of a certain height (a chart is located in the appendix at the back of this book). If the present weight falls within that range, use it for the following calculations. If the present weight falls outside of or is below the range, use the middle point of the healthy weight range as the reference weight.
- Convert the weight in pounds to kilograms (pounds divided by 2.2 equals kilograms).
- Multiply kilograms by 0.8 (**Side Note**: males 15-18 yrs. old, multiply by 0.9), to get the RDA in grams per day.

Example:

Weight = 150 lbs.

150 lbs. ÷ 2.2 lb/kg = 68 kg (rounded off)

68 kg x 0.8 g/kg = 54 g protein (rounded off)

When setting the recommended daily allowance, it is assumed that individuals are healthy and do not have abnormal metabolic needs for protein. The protein that is consumed will be of mixed quality, and the body will use the protein efficiently as it is needed.

The protein in selected foods other than protein-rich foods is as follows:

- 1 slice whole grain bread = 4 grams of protein
- ½ cup vegetables = 2 grams of protein
- 1 cup milk = 8 grams of protein
- ½ cup cooked legumes or beans = 7 grams of protein

Besides protein-rich animal foods, many other nutritious foods provide protein as well. In summary, a well balanced diet provides adequate amounts of protein for a healthy individual.

Protein and Amino Acid Supplements

In this day and age, websites, health food stores, articles in popular magazines, and books promote a wide variety of protein supplements and individual amino acids. Many individuals take these supplements for numerous reasons, most of them untested. Athletes take them in order to build or maintain more muscle. Dieters take them in order to lose fat and maintain muscle. There are many "magic pills" out on the market, all touted to help create a better, slimmer, more muscular body, but in reality it comes back to balanced nutrition and exercise.

When a balanced healthy diet is consumed, it is adequate to meet the needs of a fit and active body. At times, it may be necessary to add extra protein to the diet, but it is better to get it from a food source than from supplements. Taking a protein powder in order to consume more protein is convenient and not considerably expensive, and is something to look into. But it should not to be the main source of protein intake in the diet. Muscle work builds muscle; protein supplements do not.

In summary, a normal healthy individual is able to get the protein that the body needs to maintain or build muscle. Protein supplements and amino acids supplements are rarely required. Consuming a balanced diet and staying active will stimulate muscle growth and maintenance. Using a protein powder as a source of protein is fine, but it should not be the main source of protein in the diet. All the great technology and scientific knowledge available does not improve on the natural sources of protein which God has created for us to consume.

CHAPTER 4
About Fats

The majority of individuals are taken by surprise when informed that fat has value in a healthy diet. Only when either too much or too little fat is consumed does it affect the body in a negative way.

In fact, fat is a subset of the classes of nutrients know as lipids—compounds which contain triglycerides (fats and oils), phospholipids, and sterols. (**Side Note:** Of the lipids in food, 95 percent are fats and oils known as triglycerides, and the other 5 percent are other lipids, or phospholipids and sterols. Of the lipids that are stored in the body, 99 percent are triglycerides.)

The Breakdown of Fatty Acids and Triglycerides
Fatty Acids

Fatty acids are an organic acid—a chain of carbon atoms with hydrogen attached—that has an acid group at one end and a methyl group at the other end.

The length of most naturally occurring fatty acids contains even numbers of carbons in their chains—about 24 carbons in length. The long chain (12-24 carbons) fatty acids are found most commonly in meats and fish. Smaller amounts of medium chains (6-10 carbons) and short chains (fewer than 6 carbons) of fatty acids also occur, typically in dairy products.

The Degree of Unsaturation of Fatty Acids

Saturated fatty acids are fatty acids carrying the maximum possible number of hydrogen atoms. For example, stearic acid is a saturated fat composed of triglycerides, in which most of the fatty acids are saturated. When a fatty acid has two hydrogen atoms missing and a double bond, it is known as an unsaturated fatty acid. An unsaturated fatty acid is a fatty acid which lacks hydrogen atoms and contains at least one double bond between carbons. This includes what are known as monounsaturated fatty acids (a fatty acid that lacks two hydrogen atoms and has only one double bond between carbons), and polyunsaturated fatty acids (a fatty acid that lacks four or more hydrogen atoms and has two or more double bonds between carbons). The following is an example of oleic acid, an 18-carbon monounsaturated fatty acid and linoleic acid, an 18-carbon polyunsaturated fatty acid:

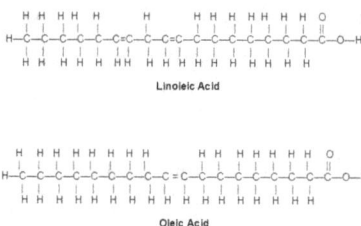

The double bond is known as the point of unsaturation of a fatty acid, where hydrogen atoms can easily be added to the structure. Therefore, a fatty acid with two hydrogen atoms missing, and a double bond is an unsaturated fatty acid.

It is important to keep in mind that all fatty acids differ, not only in the length of their chains and the degree of saturation, but in the location of their double bond as well.

The Degree of Unsaturation of Triglycerides

Triglycerides are the chief form of fat in the diet, and the major storage form of fat in the body. Triglycerides are made up of a molecule of glycerol—an alcohol composed of a three-carbon chain, which serves as the backbone—with three fatty acids attached, which are also known as triacylglycerols.

The makeup of a fatty acid—whether it is short or long, saturated or unsaturated, with its first double bond here or there—influences the characteristics of foods and the health of the body.

The degree of unsaturation of triglycerides is recognized by the following:

- **Firmness**—Unsaturation influences the firmness of fats at room temperature. Usually, the polyunsaturated vegetable oils are liquid at room temperature, and the more saturated animal fats are solid. However, not all vegetable oils are polyunsaturated. Cocoa butter, palm oil, and coconut oil are saturated, even though they are a derivative of vegetable origin. They are firmer than most vegetable oils because of their saturation, but softer than most animal fats because of their shorter carbon chains. The shorter the carbon chain, the softer the fat is at room temperature. Butter is more saturated than margarine, which is why individuals limiting their saturated fat intake use margarine.

- **Stability**—Saturation plays a role in the stability of fats. All fats can become rancid when exposed to oxygen. This is known as oxidation—the process of a substance combining with oxygen. The oxidation of unsaturated fats produces a variety of compounds that smell and taste rancid. Saturated fats are more resistant to oxidation and less likely to become rancid. Many steps are taken to keep fats from becoming rancid, including airtight packaging of foods that contain oil, the addition of antioxidants to compete for oxygen which protects the oil, and adding hydrogen molecules to foods that contain oil.

- **Hydrogenation**—Hydrogenation is a chemical process in which hydrogen molecules are added to monounsaturated or polyunsaturated fats in order to reduce the number of double bonds, making the fats more saturated (solid) and more resistant to oxidation (protecting against rancidity). Hydrogenation has two advantages: it prolongs shelf life, and it alters the texture of foods. However, foods that contain hydrogenated oils lose any of the health benefits of using unsaturated fats, and for this reason they should be avoided.

- **Trans-Fatty Acids**—Another disadvantage of foods that contain hydrogenated oils is that some of the molecules that remain unsaturated after processing change shape. When the hydrogen atoms next to the double bonds are on the same side of the carbon chain, these are known as trans-fatty acids—fatty acids with an unusual configuration around the double bond. Trans-fatty acids affect functions in the body differently, and these acids act more like saturated fats than like unsaturated fats.

In summary, the lipids in nutrition are made up of three classes: triglycerides (usually known as fats, and the primary lipids in both food and in the body), phospholipids, and sterols. The lipids that are fully loaded with hydrogen are known as saturated, and those lipids that are missing hydrogen and those that have double bonds are known as unsaturated (monounsaturated and polyunsaturated). The greater part of triglycerides contains more than one kind of fatty acid, and fatty acid saturation affects fat's physical makeup and storage properties. Hydrogenation makes unsaturated fats more saturated by changing the physical makeup, giving rise to trans-fatty acids, which alter the fatty acids and may cause serious health problems within the body.

Overview of Phospholipids and Sterols

The other two classes of lipids are the phospholipids and sterols. These make up about 5 percent of the lipids in the diet, but they are nonetheless important.

Phospholipids

Phospholipids are compounds similar to triglycerides but have a phosphate group (a phosphorus-containing salt) and choline (or another nitrogen-containing compound) in place of one of the fatty acids. The fatty acids make phospholipids soluble in fat, which allows the phosphate group to dissolve them in water. Such adaptability enables the food industry to utilize phospholipids as emulsifiers, to mix fats with water in such products as mayonnaise and candy bars.

In addition to being used by the food industry as emulsifiers, phospholipids can be found in foods naturally. The best-known phospholipid occurring naturally in foods is lecithin—a compound of glycerol which is attached to two fatty acids, a phosphate group, and a choline molecule. The best food sources in which lecithin can be found are eggs, liver, soybeans, wheat germ, and peanuts.

Lecithin and other phospholipids are an important element of cell membranes. Because phospholipids can dissolve in both fat and water, they are able to help lipids move back and forth across the cell membranes into the watery fluids on both sides. They allow fat-soluble substances, including vitamins and hormones, to pass easily in and out of cells. Also, phospholipids act as emulsifiers in the body, helping to keep fats suspended in the blood and body fluids.

In summary, phospholipids (including lecithin) have a unique chemical structure which allows them to be soluble in both fat and water. The food industry makes great use of phospholipids as emulsifiers. In the body, phospholipids are an important part of cell membranes.

Sterols

Sterols are compounds composed of carbon, hydrogen, and oxygen atoms arranged in rings, with any variety of side chains attached. The most well-known sterol is cholesterol.

Sterols are found in foods from both plants and animals. However, the sterols from animal sources—meat, eggs, fish, poultry, and dairy products—contain cholesterol.

Many significantly important body compounds are made up of sterols. Among them are bile, the sex hormones, the adrenal hormones, vitamin D, and cholesterol itself. Cholesterol in the body is able to serve as the initial material for the synthesis of these compounds, or to serve as a structural element of cell membranes. Contrary to popular belief, cholesterol is not a villain waiting in some evil foods to cause the body to have health problems. It is a compound that the body makes and uses all the time. Cholesterol's harmful effects occur when it forms deposits in the artery walls. These deposits can lead to heart disease, which can cause heart attacks and strokes.

In summary, sterols (including cholesterol) have a multiple-ring structure which is different from all other lipids. Certain body compounds are made up of sterols, and only animal-derived foods contain cholesterol.

Digestion and Absorption of Fats

It is estimated that each day the GI tract receives about 50-100 grams of triglycerides, 4-8 grams of phospholipids, and 300-450 milligrams of cholesterol. The body has the challenge of digesting and absorbing these lipids. Because fats are hydrophobic—they tend to separate from the watery fluids of the GI tract—and the enzymes for digesting fats are hydrophilic—water soluble. The challenge is how the body mixes the fats into the watery fluids and is able to digest them.

The objective of fat digestion is to break down triglycerides into small molecules that the body is able to absorb and use—specifically, monoglycerides (molecules of glycerol with one fatty acid attached), fatty acids, and glycerol.

Digestion and Absorption Starts in the Mouth

Fat digestion starts slowly in the mouth, with the hard fats beginning to melt when they reach body temperature. Once this occurs, a salivary gland at the base of the tongue releases an enzyme called lingual lipase, which plays a small role in fat digestion in adults, but an active role in infants. (**Side Note**: in infants, this enzyme efficiently digests the short- and medium-chain fatty acids found in milk.)

The Stomach

In a calm stomach, fat floats as a layer above the other components of swallowed food. However, the muscle contractions of the stomach and the periodic emptying of chyme (the semi-liquid mass of partly digested food) through the pyloric sphincter churn which mixes the stomach contents. This action helps to expose the fat which is attack by the gastric enzymes called lipase. It works mainly on short-chain fatty acids. Very little of fat digestion takes place in the stomach; most of this action takes place in the small intestine.

The Small Intestine

Once the fat enters the small intestine, it triggers the release of the hormone cholecystokinin (CCK), which signals the gallbladder to release its stores of bile. (**Side Note**: The liver produces bile acids from cholesterol, and the gallbladder stores the bile until it is needed.)

At one end of each bile acid are side chains of amino acids or units of protein that are attracted to water. At the other end is a sterol that is attracted to fat. This unique structure allows bile to act as an emulsifier, drawing fat molecules into the surrounding watery fluids. The fats are fully digested as they encounter the lipase enzymes that are released from the pancreas and small intestine.

The majority of the breakdown of triglycerides occurs in the small intestine. The major fat-digesting enzymes, pancreatic lipases, are active during this particular process of digestion. These enzymes remove one, then the other, of each triglyceride's outer fatty acids, leaving only a monoglyceride. Sporadically, enzymes remove all three fatty acids, leaving a free molecule of glycerol.

Phospholipids are broken down in a similar manner—that is, their fatty acids are removed by enzymes. They are left with two fatty acids and fragmented phospholipids, which are then absorbed.

Sterols are broken down and are able to be absorbed as is; usually no fatty acids remain.

Bile's Routes

After the bile has entered the small intestine and has emulsified the fat, it has two likely objectives. Most of the bile is reabsorbed from the intestine and recycled. However, some of the bile can be trapped by dietary fibers in the large intestine and carried out of the body in the feces.

Absorption into the Bloodstream

The small molecules of digested triglycerides (glycerol and short- and medium-chain fatty acids) are diffused easily into the intestinal cells and are absorbed directly into the bloodstream. The larger molecules (the monoglycerides and long-chain fatty acids) come together into circular complexes known as micelles—tiny circular complexes of emulsified fat that arise during digestion. Each carries about a dozen molecules of bile and fatty acids and/or monoglycerides. This arrangement allows solubility in the watery digestive fluids and transportation to the intestinal cells. Upon entrance into the intestinal cells, the micelles diffuse. Once inside, the monoglycerides and long-chain fatty acids are reassembled into new triglycerides.

Therefore, inside the intestinal cells, the newly made triglycerides and the other large lipids or fats (cholesterol and phospholipids) are packed into transport vessels known as chylomicrons—a type of lipoprotein that transports lipids from the intestinal cells to the rest of the body. The intestinal cells release the chylomicrons into the lymphatic system. The chylomicrons slide along through the lymph until they reach a point of entry into the bloodstream. The blood then carries these lipids to the rest of the body.

In summary, the body formulates special arrangements to digest and absorb lipids. It allows the emulsifier bile to make lipids accessible to the fat-digesting lipases, which dismantle triglycerides (mostly into monoglycerides and fatty acids) for absorption by the intestinal cells. The intestinal cells assemble newly absorbed lipids into chylomicrons—lipid packages with protein escorts—for transport, so that cells all over the body are able to select needed lipids from the bloodstream.

Lipid Transport

Chylomicrons are only one of several clusters of lipids and proteins that are used as transport vessels for fats. As a group, these transport vessels are known as lipoproteins—clusters of lipids associated with proteins which serve as transport vessels for lipids in the lymph and blood. They efficiently solve the body's challenge of transporting fatty materials through the watery bloodstream. The body is able to make four main types of lipoproteins, distinguished by their size and density. Each contains different kinds and amounts of proteins and lipids; the more proteins, the higher the density, and the more lipids, the lower the density. The four types of lipoproteins are:

- **Chylomicrons**—Chylomicrons are the largest and least dense of the lipoproteins. They transport lipids derived from the diet (mostly triglycerides) from the intestine to the rest of the body via the bloodstream. Cells throughout the body remove lipids from the chylomicrons as they pass by, and the chylomicrons get smaller and smaller. Special protein receptors on the membranes of the liver cells distinguish and remove the chylomicron remnants from the blood. After collecting the remnants, the liver cells dismantle them and promptly reassemble the pieces into new triglycerides.

- **VLDL (Very-Low-Density Lipoproteins)**—VLDL is the type of lipoprotein made primarily by liver cells to transport lipids to various tissues in the body. These are composed mainly of triglycerides. As the VLDL pass through the body, cells remove triglycerides, causing the VLDL to shrink. When the VLDL loses triglycerides, the proportion of lipids shifts and the lipoprotein eventually becomes a low-density lipoprotein. This is why LDL contains few triglycerides but is loaded with cholesterol.

- **LDL (Low-Density Lipoproteins)**—LDL is the type of lipoprotein derived from very-low-density lipoproteins when cells remove triglycerides from them. These are composed mainly of cholesterol. The LDL flows throughout the body, making their contents available to the cells of all tissues—muscles, including the heart muscle, fat stores, the mammary glands, and others. These cells take triglycerides, cholesterol, and phospholipids to build new membranes, make hormones or other compounds, or store for later use. The special LDL receptors on the liver cells work hard to control the blood cholesterol concentrations by removing LDL from the circulation.

- **HDL (High-Density Lipoproteins)**—HDL is the type of lipoprotein that transports cholesterol back to the liver from the cells, and HDL is composed mainly of protein.

In summary, the liver is where lipids, along with proteins, are packaged into lipoproteins for transport throughout the body. All four types of lipoproteins carry all classes of lipids, but chylomicrons are the largest and the highest in triglycerides; VLDL are smaller; LDL are smaller still and are high in cholesterol; and HDL are the smallest and are rich in protein.

Lipids in the Body

The bloodstream carries lipids to various sites throughout the body. Once they arrive at their destinations, the lipids do their work of providing energy, insulating against extreme temperatures, protecting against shock, and building cell structures.

Roles of Triglycerides in the Body

Triglycerides—either from food or the body's fat stores—provide the body with energy. When a woman goes out for a morning ten-mile run, her breakfast's triglycerides provide the fuel to keep her moving. If a man loses his appetite for some reason, his stored triglycerides fuel much of the body's work until he can eat again.

Fats are essential for insulating the body and act as shock absorbers, supporting and cushioning the vital organs. Fat is a poor conductor of heat, so the layer of fat beneath the skin helps keep the body warm.

Fats help the body use its two energy nutrients—carbohydrates and proteins—efficiently. When fat fragments combine with glucose fragments during energy metabolism, the fat helps spare protein and provides energy so that protein can be used for other important tasks.

Roles of Essential Fatty Acids

The body needs fatty acids, and it is able to make all but two of them—linoleic acid (omega-6) and linolenic acid (omega-3). These two fatty acids need to be supplied by the diet, and are therefore referred to as essential fatty acids—fatty acids required by the body, but not made by the body in amounts sufficient to meet all the body's needs.

The cells within the body do not possess the enzymes to make any of the omega-6 or omega-3 fatty acids from scratch; nor are they able to convert an omega-6 fatty acid to an omega-3 fatty acid, or vice versa. The most effective way to maintain the body's supply of omega-6 and omega-3 fatty acids is to obtain them directly from foods—particularly from vegetable oils, seeds, nuts, and fish.

Linoleic Acid

Linoleic acid is the main member of the omega-6 family. When given linoleic acid, the body is able to make other members of the omega-6 family—such as arachidonic acid, a polyunsaturated fatty acid. This particular fatty acid contains 20 carbons and 4 double bonds (20:4), and is synthesized from linoleic acid. If a linoleic acid deficiency develops, arachidonic acid, and any other fatty acids that are derived from linoleic acid, would become essential and need to be obtained from the diet. Usually, vegetable oils and meats supply enough omega-6 fatty acids to meet the body's needs.

Linolenic Acid

Linolenic acid is the main member of the omega-3 family. Like linoleic acid, this acid cannot be made in the body and needs to be supplied by foods. When given linolenic acid, the body is able to make other members of the omega-3 family—such as EPA (eicosapentaenoic acid) and DHA (docosahexaenoic acid). Eicosapentaenoic acid contains 20 carbons and 5 double bonds (20:5), while docosahexaenoic acid contains 22 carbons and 6 double bonds (22:6). Omega-3 fatty acids are essential for normal growth and development, and they may play an important role in the prevention and treatment of heart disease, hypertension, arthritis, and cancer.

Fatty Acid Deficiencies

Essential fatty acids should make up at least 3 percent of the day's energy intake, and most diets meet this minimum requirement. However, deficiencies do develop, and the most widely known essential fatty acid deficiencies are found in people with chronic intestinal diseases. Deficiency symptoms include growth retardation, reproductive failure, skin lesions, kidney and liver disorders, and subtle neurological and visual problems.

In summary, linoleic acid (omega-6) and linolenic acid (omega-3) are essential nutrients. Not only do they serve as structural parts of cell membranes, they make powerful compounds that help to regulate blood pressure, blood clot formation, and the immune response to injury and infection. Deficiencies are not common, but are apparent in those who have chronic intestinal diseases. Triglycerides which reside in the body play the following important parts:

- Provide an energy reserve when stored in the body's fat tissue
- Insulate against temperature extremes
- Protect organs against shock
- Help the body use carbohydrates and protein efficiently

Lipid Metabolism

The bloodstream delivers triglycerides to the cells, and it is either used as a source of energy or stored as fat. The following points are an overview of how the cells store and release energy from fat:

- **Fat Stored as Fat**—Triglycerides produced by the body, similar to fat in foods, serve the body primarily as a source of fuel. Fat provides more than twice the energy of carbohydrates and proteins, making it an exceedingly efficient form of energy for storage. The body's fat stores have a virtually unlimited capacity because of the special cells known as adipose tissue—the body's fat tissue, which consists of masses of fat-storing cells. Different from most of the body's cells, which can store only limited amounts of fat, the fat cells of adipose tissue readily take up and store fat. Adipose cells have an enzyme on their surfaces—lipoprotein lipase—that captures circulating triglycerides from lipoproteins passing by in the bloodstream after a meal. This enzyme breaks down the triglycerides into fatty acids and monoglycerides and distributes them into the cells. Once inside the cells, other enzymes reassemble the pieces back into triglycerides for storage. Triglycerides tend to be packed tightly together within the adipose cells, storing a lot of energy in a rather small area.

- **Making Fat from Carbohydrate or Protein**—Fatty acids can be made from two-carbon fragments derived from carbohydrates or proteins. Glucose is able to be converted to body fat, because enzymes break the glucose into fragments and then combines them to make long-chain fatty acids. Enzymes can also convert some of the components of certain amino acids to fatty acids. Still, the food source from which the body is most easily able to store fat is from fat itself.

- **Making Fat from Fat**—In order to convert foods to body fat, the body breaks the food down, absorbs the food, and through a simple process puts the food together again in storage. It takes relatively little energy to break down fats, and it takes more energy to break down carbohydrates and proteins. Each conversion requires energy, and it costs less (energy-wise) to store dietary fats as body fat than to convert and store dietary carbohydrates and proteins as body fat.

- **Using Fat for Energy**—Fat supplies about 60 percent of the body's ongoing energy needs during rest, but during prolonged periods of light to moderately intense exercise or extended bouts of food deprivation, fat stores may make a slightly greater contribution to energy needs. This is because when cells need energy, an enzyme known as hormone-sensitive lipase—an enzyme inside adipose cells that responds to the body's need for fuel—breaks down triglycerides so that their glycerol and fatty acids escape into the bloodstream and become available to other cells as fuel. Cells anywhere in the body that lack energy can then capture these compounds and take them through a chain of chemical reactions in order to yield energy.

In summary, the body is designed to be able to store unlimited amounts of excess fat, and this body fat is then used for energy when needed. The liver can convert excess carbohydrates and proteins into fat as well. For maximum efficiency, it is important for a carbohydrate to be present during fat breakdown; without carbohydrates, fats break down into ketone bodies.

Health Effects and Intake of Lipids

Out of all the nutrients, fat is most often linked to chronic diseases. A diet that is high in saturated fats and hydrogenated oils raises the risk of heart disease, some types of cancer, hypertension, diabetes, and obesity.

Heart Disease

Most individuals realize that elevated blood cholesterol is a major risk factor for heart disease, better known as cardiovascular disease. Cholesterol, when it accumulates in the arteries, restricts the blood flow and raises the blood pressure. The consequences can be deadly if gone undetected. The mainstream media tells people how to cut the cholesterol in their diets, but what most individuals do not realize is that food cholesterol does not necessarily raise blood cholesterol as dramatically as saturated fat does.

Remember that LDL cholesterol increases the risk of heart disease, and most often implicated in the raising of LDL cholesterol are the saturated fats. Not all saturated fatty acids have the same cholesterol-raising effect, but most notable among the saturated fatty acids that raise blood cholesterol are lauric, myristic, and palmitic acids. In contrast, stearic acid does not appear to raise blood cholesterol, but it may similarly increase the risk of heart disease. Additionally, these saturated fatty acids typically appear together in the same foods, making such distinctions impractical or almost impossible when planning the diet. Common sources of stearic acid and other saturated fats include red meat, high-fat milk products, and chocolate.

Trans-fatty acids—even the monounsaturated ones—alter blood cholesterol the same way that some saturated fats tend to do; they raise

LDL and lower HDL cholesterol. Replacing both saturated fats and trans-fats with monounsaturated and polyunsaturated fats may be the most effective strategy in preventing heart disease.

It has been found that omega-3 polyunsaturated fatty acids are helpful in lowering blood cholesterol and preventing heart disease. A diet low in both saturated fat and trans-fats, in combination with polyunsaturated fats, will help lower the risk of heart disease.

Cancer

Although the link between dietary fats and cancer is not as clear as that of heart disease, it is suggested that an association between the kinds of fat and the total amount of fat may contribute to some types of cancer. It is thought that dietary fat does not seem to initiate the development of cancer, but dietary fat can promote cancer once it has arisen.

The relationship between dietary fat and the risk of cancer differs for various kinds of cancer. For example, in the case of breast cancer, evidence has been inconclusive. But in the case of prostate cancer, there seems to be a strong evidence of association with fat.

The relationship between dietary fat and the risk of cancer differs for various kinds of fats as well. The association between fat and cancer appears to be mainly from saturated fats, primarily those found in red meat, high-fat milk products, and highly processed foods.

Obesity

Individuals who tend to eat a very high-fat diet store body fat efficiently and have more body fat than they will ever need, even during dire circumstances. To limit the possibility of obesity, it is vital that individuals consume a balanced diet—one that appropriately satisfies hunger and provides enough energy for bodily functions and activities.

In summary, a diet high in excessive dietary fat contributes to heart disease, some types of cancer, obesity, and other major health problems.

Intake of Fats

Triglycerides naturally occur in certain proteins derived from animals, such as meat, fish, poultry, and eggs, as well as in certain carbohydrates derived from plants, such as avocados and coconuts. Another important fact about triglycerides is that they bear the four fat-soluble vitamins—A, D, E, and K.

Some fat in a healthy diet is essential for overall good health. But too much fat, especially saturated fat, increases the risk for chronic diseases. Dietary fat recommendations include the following:

- Reduce total fat intake to 30 percent or less of energy intake
- Reduce saturated fat intake to less than 10 percent of energy intake
- Reduce cholesterol intake to less than 300 milligrams daily

In order to meet dietary fat recommendations, many individuals need to reduce their fat intakes. The following are tips to help lower total fat intake and encourage the consumption of healthier choices.

- **Reduce Total Fat Intake**—Fat accounts for a lot of the energy in foods, and removing the excessive fat from foods cuts the energy intake significantly. To eliminate fat as a seasoning and in cooking, remove the fat from the high-fat foods. It is easy to replace high-fat foods with low-fat alternatives and accompany this with an emphasis on vegetables, fruits, and grains.

- **Reduce Saturated and Trans-Fat Intake**—In the diets of most individuals, fats from animal sources are the main source of saturated fat, although some vegetable fats (coconut and palm) provide smaller amounts of saturated fats. Selecting poultry or fish and nonfat dairy products helps to lower the total saturated fat intake and heart disease risk. Limiting the intake of trans-fatty acids (which include partially hydrogenated oils) can lower the risk of heart disease.

- **Reduce Cholesterol Intake**—Cholesterol is found mainly in animal products. Therefore, eating less fat from meat, eggs, and dairy products will help lower dietary cholesterol (as well as saturated fat intake). For most individuals, it is more effective to limit the saturated fat intake than it is to limit the cholesterol intake. For example, eggs are a valued part of the diet because they are inexpensive, useful in cooking, and a good source of high-quality protein. However, one egg contains just over 200 milligrams of cholesterol, all of it in the yolk. But the yolk also contains lethicin, which aids in lowering cholesterol. Some research suggests that eating one egg a day is not a health threat for otherwise healthy individuals.

- **Balance Omega-3 and Omega-6 Intakes**—In order to obtain the right balance between omega-3 and omega-6 acids, most individuals need to consume more fish and less meat. It is possible to get omega-3 acids from oils (flaxseed, canola, walnut, wheat germ, and soy bean), nuts (butternuts, walnuts, and soybean kernels), and vegetables (soybeans). And it is possible to get omega-6 acids from vegetable oils (corn, sunflower, safflower, soybean, and cottonseed). In addition, other foods are being developed to help consumers improve their omega-3 and omega-6 intake. Many types of bread, cereals, and other products have sources of omega-3 and omega-6 added to them nowadays.

- **Select Lean Meats and Nonfat Milks**—Many foods that contain fat, saturated fat, and cholesterol in high levels—such as meats, eggs, and dairy products—also provide high-quality protein and important vitamins and minerals. They can be included in a healthful diet when an individual selects lean and nonfat products and prepares them in a way that reduces the total fat, saturated fat, and cholesterol.

- **Use Fats and Oils Sparingly**—Learn to practice moderation when using fats and oils such as butter, mayonnaise, and salad dressings. These may taste good, but offer little nourishment and a lot of extra fat.

- **Beware of Hidden Fat**—Hidden fat is less apparent than visible fat, such as butter, oil in salad dressing, or the fat trimmed from meat. Hidden fat is the marbling of a steak or is in foods like nuts, cheese, avocados, and olives. These are considered healthy fats and should, like all foods, be consumed in moderation. On the other hand, fried foods (potato chips, French fries, and many others) contain abundant amounts of fat. Many baked goods are high in fat, including pie crusts, pastries, crackers, biscuits, doughnuts, cookies, and cakes. Keep invisible fats in mind when making healthful food selections.

- **Choose Wisely**—It is best to choose a diet that is low in saturated fat and cholesterol, while consuming a moderate intake of healthy fats. Fat is needed in a healthy diet for the body to function and operate optimally. Do not forgo fats altogether, and make sure the kinds of fats that are consumed are healthful fats.

- **Eat Plenty of Vegetables, Fruits, and Grains**—Choosing a variety of fruits, vegetables, and grains will aid in lowering total fat intake. Vegetables and fruits naturally contain no fat, and most grains contain only trace amounts. It has been shown that a low-fat diet rich in vegetables, fruits, and grains offers an abundance of vitamin C, folate, vitamin A, and dietary fiber— all important in supporting good health. Such a diet protects against diseases by reducing fat and increasing healthful nutrients.

- **Read Food Labels**—Labels on food products list total fat, saturated fat, and cholesterol. Since each food package provides information for a single serving and serving sizes are standardized, consumers can easily compare similar products and choose the most beneficial product to consume. It is a good idea to read the ingredients in a product to see if it contains any trans-fats from hydrogenated fats. If hydrogenated fats are listed more than twice in the ingredients, it is best to not consume the product.

In summary, some fat is necessary for overall health. It is best to limit total fat intake to 30 percent. It is recommended to consume more monounsaturated and polyunsaturated fats—particularly omega-3 and omega-6 fatty acids—from foods in the diet and not from supplements. The key is not deprivation but moderation. Appreciate the energy and enjoyment that fat provides but take care not to exceed your needs!

CHAPTER 5
About Vitamins and Minerals

A combination of 30 vitamins and minerals is required for overall good health. For the most part, your body can't make vitamins or minerals, so these must be supplied from the consumption of a variety of foods. Vitamins certainly support nutritional health, but they do not cure all ills. Furthermore, vitamin supplements do not offer the many benefits that come from vitamin-rich foods.

The role of vitamins in supporting optimal health extends far beyond preventing vitamin-deficiency diseases. Actually, some of the credit given to low-fat diets in preventing disease in reality belongs to the vitamins that diets rich in vegetables, fruits, and grains deliver.

Vitamins differ from carbohydrates, fats, and proteins in the following ways:

- **Structure**—Vitamins are individual units and are not linked together (as are molecules of glucose, fatty acids, or amino acids).
- **Function**—Vitamins do not yield usable energy when broken down, and they assist the enzymes that release energy from carbohydrates, fats, and proteins.
- **Food Contents**—The amounts of vitamins individuals ingest daily from foods and the amount required are measured in micrograms or milligrams, rather than in grams.

Vitamins are similar to the energy-yielding nutrients in that they are vital to life, are organic, and are available from foods.

An Overview of Vitamins

From vitamin A to vitamin K, these nutrients in minute quantities facilitate hundreds of biochemical reactions in the body. Vitamins also act as regulators which oversee processes like bone growth and the maintenance of healthy skin. Vitamins are vitally important. Without them, it would be difficult to process the carbohydrates the body needs for stamina, the body's protein metabolism would fall apart, and the body would slowly degenerate—becoming anemic, weak, unable to think clearly, and would eventually die.

Bioavailability

The availability of vitamins from foods depends on two factors:

- The quality provided by food
- The amount absorbed and used by the body

Researchers analyze foods in order to determine their vitamin content and publish the results. Determining the bioavailability—which refers to the rate at and the extent to which a nutrient is absorbed and used—of a vitamin is a more complex task than it seems, because it depends on many factors. They are as follows:

- Efficiency of digestion and time of transit through the GI tract
- Previous nutrient intake and nutrition status
- Other foods consumed at the same time
- Method of food preparation (raw, cooked, or processed)
- Source of the nutrient (synthetic, fortified, or naturally occurring)

All these factors are taken into consideration when experts estimate the recommended intakes for each vitamin.

Precursors

A number of vitamins are available from foods in inactive forms known as precursors—substances that precede others—with regard to vitamins and compounds that can be converted into active vitamins. Once inside the body, the precursor is changed chemically into an active form of the vitamin.

Organic Nature

Being an organic substance, vitamins can be destroyed and left unable to perform their rightful duties. They must be handled with care during storage and cooking. Extensive heating may destroy many of the important vitamins in food. Ways to minimize nutrient loss in foods are as follows:

- Refrigerate most vegetables and fruits
- Store vegetables and fruits that have been cut in airtight containers
- Store juices in closed containers after opening
- Rinse vegetables and fruits lightly before cutting
- Avoid high temperatures and long cooking times
- Add vegetables to water after it has come to a boil

Solubility

Carbohydrates and proteins are hydrophilic and lipids are hydrophobic, and vitamins divide along the same lines. The hydrophilic, better known as the water-soluble vitamins, are the B vitamins and vitamin C. The hydrophobic, or fat-soluble vitamins, are A, D, E, and K.

It has been noted that solubility is apparent in the food sources of the different vitamins, and it tends to affect their absorption, transport, storage, and excretion by the body. The water-soluble vitamins are found in the watery portion of foods, and the fat-soluble vitamins are found in the fats and oils of foods. Once absorbed, the water-soluble vitamins travel directly into the bloodstream. The fat-soluble vitamins must enter the lymph, and from there travel to the bloodstream. Upon reaching the cells, water-soluble vitamins circulate freely in the water-filled portions of the body, and fat-soluble vitamins are stored in fatty tissues and in the liver until needed.

Since the body stores fat-soluble vitamins, they can be eaten in large amounts once in a while and still be able to meet the body's needs over time. Water-soluble vitamins are kept for varying periods in the body. A single day's exclusion from the diet does not bring on a deficiency, but it is important that water-soluble vitamins be eaten more regularly than fat-soluble vitamins. The following are the water-soluble and fat-soluble vitamin groups:

Water-Soluble Vitamins:

- Vitamin B1 (Thiamin)
- Vitamin B2 (Riboflavin)

- Vitamin B3 (Niacin)
- Vitamin B5 (Pantothenic acid)
- Vitamin B6 (Pyridoxine)
- Biotin
- Folate
- Vitamin C

Fat-Soluble Vitamins:

- Vitamin A
- Vitamin D
- Vitamin E
- Vitamin K

Toxicity

Many individuals have the idea that if getting vitamins is important, they should begin taking vitamin supplements, assuming that more is better. An inadequate intake of vitamins can cause damage, but so can an excessive intake. Therefore, vitamins can be both essential and damaging, which is true of most nutrients.

In summary, vitamins are essential nutrients that are needed in small amounts in a healthy diet—both to prevent deficiency diseases and to support optimal health. The tables that follow summarize the difference between the water-soluble and fat-soluble vitamins:

Water-Soluble Vitamins B Vitamins and Vitamin C

- **Absorption**: Directly into the bloodstream

- **Transport**: Travel freely

- **Storage**: Circulate freely in water-filled parts of the body

- **Excretion**: Kidneys detect and remove excess in the urine

- **Toxicity**: Possible to reach toxic levels when consumed from supplements

- **Requirements**: Needed in numerous doses (for example, every one to three days)

Fat-Soluble Vitamins Vitamins A, D, E, and K

- **Absorption**: Through the lymph and then into the bloodstream

- **Transport**: Requires protein carriers

- **Storage**: Stored in cells associated with fat

- **Excretion**: Not readily excreted and tend to remain in fat storage sites

- **Toxicity**: Likely to reach toxic levels when consumed from supplements.

- **Requirements**: Needed in periodic doses (for example, once a week, or even once a month)

Vitamins in the Body

Once the digestive tract absorbs the vitamins from a meal, along with the carbohydrates, proteins, fats, and minerals, it is time for these substances to begin working in the body. For the most part, the water-soluble vitamins move quickly throughout the body, doing their job, processing the other nutrients from a meal. The body does not have the ability to store these vitamins for later use, so within 24-48 hours, the water-soluble vitamins turn over, meaning they are broken down into useful elements or excreted in brightly colored urine within eight hours after taking the vitamin pill. The excess water-soluble vitamins spill into the urine and go unused.

On the other hand, fat-soluble vitamins are not disposed of as quickly, and can be stored for later use in various parts throughout the body, particularly the liver. For example, the liver has about a one- to two-year supply of vitamin A. Because of this storage ability, the body is able to go for extended periods of time when the diet supplies a poor amount of vitamin A, without seeing the ill effects of a deficiency. Conversely, water-soluble vitamin deficiencies show up about 40-60 days when the diet supplies a poor amount.

In summary, it is important to know that each vitamin has a unique role in the body, and that each works with the food that is consumed to maintain health.

Vitamins in Food

Despite the wide availability of vitamins, many individuals fall short of the daily requirement due to poor food choices and habits. In general, when foods like fruits, vegetables, and whole grains are processed in any way—peeled, cooked, or separated—vitamin content is lowered. For better vitamin nutrients, individuals need to include unprocessed foods. For example, when sliced vegetables are soaked in water, many of the water-soluble vitamins are likely to leach out, lowering the energy of the vitamins' content. To get the most nutrition from foods that are consumed, follow these simple guidelines:

- When preparing vegetables for cooking, cut them into larger pieces for better vitamin retention
- When cooking vegetables, steam or microwave rather than boil them, in order to prevent leaching into cooking water
- Store fruits and vegetables whole instead of in pieces
- Keep fruit juices in airtight containers and freeze them when possible

In summary, eating a wide variety of foods ensures sufficient intake of vitamins, just as it does with minerals.

A List of Vitamins from A to Z

Vitamin A

Function: Necessary for normal vision; maintains structure and function of mucous membranes; aids growth of bones, teeth, and skin.

Food Source: Yellow-orange vegetables and dark fruits; dark-green leafy vegetables; fortified milk; eggs; liver.

Thiamin (B-1)

Function: Necessary for carbohydrate metabolism; helps maintain healthy nervous system.

Food Source: Pork; liver; whole grain and enriched grain products; beans; nuts.

Riboflavin (B-2)

Function: Needed for carbohydrate, protein, and fat metabolism; healthy skin.

Food Source: Dairy products; whole grain and enriched grain products.

Niacin (B-3)

Function: Needed for carbohydrate, protein, and fat metabolism; nervous system function; for oxygen use by cells.

Food Source: Meats; fish; poultry; eggs; whole grain products; nuts.

Pyridoxine (B-6)

Function: Needed for protein metabolism; for normal growth.

Food Source: Meats; fish; poultry; beans; grains; green leafy vegetables.

Folate

Function: necessary for red blood cell development; for tissue growth and repair.

Food Source: Green leafy vegetables; oranges; beans; liver.

Cyanocobalamin (B-12)

Function: Needed for new tissue growth; red blood cells; nervous system; skin.

Food Source: meat; fish; poultry; dairy products.

Biotin

Function: Needed for normal metabolism of carbohydrates, proteins, and fats.

Food Source: Widespread in foods—whole grain products; fish; meat; dairy products.

Pantothenic Acid (B-5)

Function: Needed for normal metabolism of carbohydrates, proteins, and fats.

Food Source: Widespread in foods—whole grain products; meats; vegetables; eggs.

Vitamin C

Function: Needed for building collagen; healthy gums; teeth; blood vessels.

Food Source: Citrus fruits; peppers; cabbage family vegetables; strawberries; tomatoes.

Vitamin D

Function: Needed for calcium absorption; for proper growth of bones and teeth.

Food Source: Sunlight; fortified dairy products; eggs; fish; liver.

Vitamin E

Function: Acts as an antioxidant; protects cells from damage.

Food Source: Vegetables oils; green leafy vegetables; wheat germ; whole grain products.

Vitamin K

Function: Aids in blood clotting.

Food Source: Cabbage family vegetables; green leafy vegetables.

An Overview of Minerals

Like vitamins, minerals play an important role in supporting optimal health, which extends far beyond preventing deficiency diseases. They give the body shape by providing structure to the bones and teeth. Minerals also keep the body's pH (acid level) and water in balance.

Minerals are normally grouped into two categories:

- Major Minerals
- Trace Minerals

The distinction between the major and trace minerals does not reflect the importance of one group over the other—all minerals are vital.

An Overview of Major Minerals

The major minerals are so named because they are present and are needed in larger amounts in the body. The trace minerals are so named because they are present and are needed in relatively small amounts in the body. The following are points that relate to the tasks of the major minerals:

- **Inorganic Elements**—Different from vitamins, which easily get destroyed, minerals are inorganic elements that always retain their chemical identity. Once minerals enter the body, they remain there until excreted. They are not broken down and changed into anything else. For example, iron may temporarily combine with other charged elements in salts, but it is always iron. Also, minerals cannot be destroyed by heat, air, acid, or mixing. As a result, little care is needed to preserve minerals in food preparation. In fact, the ash from food that has been burned contains all the minerals that were in the food originally. However, minerals can be lost from food when they leach into water that is then poured down the drain.

- **The Body's Use of Minerals**—Minerals again differ from vitamins in the amounts the body is able to absorb and in the extent to which they are to be specially handled. For example, some minerals, such as potassium, are easily absorbed into the bloodstream, transported freely, and readily excreted by the kidneys, much like the water-soluble vitamins. Other minerals, such as calcium, are more like fat-soluble vitamins, in that they need to have carriers to be absorbed and transported. Like the fat-soluble vitamins, minerals taken in excess can be toxic.

- **Variable Bioavailability**—The bioavailability—the rate at and the extent to which a nutrient is absorbed and used—of minerals varies. A number of foods contain binders which combine chemically with minerals, preventing their absorption and excreting them out of the body with other wastes. Binders include phytates, which are found primarily in legumes and grains, and oxalates, which are present in rhubarb and spinach, among other food. These kinds of foods actually contain more minerals than the body receives for use from them.

- **Nutrient Interactions**—Certain minerals can affect another's absorption, metabolism, and excretion. For example, the interactions between sodium and calcium cause both to be excreted when sodium intakes are high. Phosphorus binds with magnesium in the GI tract, which limits magnesium absorption when phosphorus intakes are high. Of course, these are just two examples of interactions involving minerals. (**Side Note:** It is important to note that often an excess of one mineral creates an inadequacy of another mineral, and that supplements—not foods—are most often the cause.)

- **Varied Role**—The major minerals help to maintain the body's fluid balance described earlier. However, sodium, chloride, and potassium are the most notable in that role.

In summary, the major minerals are found in larger quantities in the body, while the trace minerals occur in smaller amounts. Minerals are inorganic elements that retain their chemical identities, and they usually receive special handling and regulation in the body. Minerals may bind with other substances or interact with other minerals, thus limiting their absorption.

An Overview of Trace Minerals

The trace minerals are so named because they are present, and needed, in relatively small amounts in the body. These minerals are less important than the major minerals or any other nutrients. However, each of the trace minerals performs a vital role, and a deficiency of any of them may be fatal, or an excess of many is equally deadly. Surprisingly, an individual's diet normally supplies just enough of these minerals to maintain health. The following are points that relate to the tasks of the trace minerals:

- **Sources**—The trace mineral makeup of foods depends on the soil and water composition, as well as on how foods are processed. Plus, many factors in the diet and within the body affect the minerals bioavailability—the rate at and the extent to which a nutrient is absorbed and used. Again, high-quality food sources for each of the trace minerals, just like those for other nutrients, would include a wide variety of foods, especially unprocessed, whole foods.

- **Deficiencies**—It seems that deficiencies of the better-known minerals are easy to recognize. Others may be harder to diagnose, and for all minerals, mild deficiencies are very easy to overlook. The most common result of a deficiency is failure to grow and thrive, for the minerals are active in all the body systems—the GI tract, cardiovascular system, blood, muscles, bones, and central nervous system.

- **Toxicities**—A few of the trace minerals are toxic at intakes not far above the estimated requirements. This is why it is important not to habitually exceed the upper level of the recommended intakes. A lot of vitamin-mineral supplements contain trace minerals, which makes it easy for users to exceed their needs. Individuals who take supplements must be aware of the possible dangers, and select supplements that do not contain more than 100 percent of the daily value. It is easier and safer to meet nutrient needs without causing toxicity by eating a variety of foods than by taking an assortment of pills.

- **Interactions**—There are interactions among the trace minerals, and these often lead to nutrient imbalances, because an excess of one nutrient may cause a deficiency of another. For example, a slight manganese overload may aggravate an iron deficiency, which makes the body vulnerable to lead poisoning. Thus, a deficiency of one may open the door for another to cause a toxic reaction. Another interaction is that a good food source of one nutrient may be a poor food source of another, and factors that enhance the actions of some trace minerals may hinder others. For example, meats are a good source of iron, but a poor source of calcium. And vitamin C enhances the absorption of iron but hinders that of copper. Research on trace minerals is active, which means that there is still more to learn about them.

In summary, even though the body uses only tiny amounts of the trace minerals, they are vital to health. Since such small amounts are required, the trace minerals can be toxic at levels far above the estimated requirements, which is something that supplement users should take into consideration. But like all other nutrients, the trace minerals are best obtained by eating a variety of whole foods.

Minerals in the Body

Minerals make their way through the body along with carbohydrates, proteins, and fats from a meal. However, depending on which mineral it is, only 5-60 percent of it actually becomes part of the body. Physical properties inherent in a particular food are largely the cause for the poor absorption rate. For example, the fiber in whole grains, tannins in coffee and tea, and oxalate found in spinach and other vegetables all inhibit to a point, but do not prevent iron from entering the body.

Once the minerals enter the bloodstream, they quickly move through the watery parts of the body and end up in every cell to perform their vital task. The body continually loses minerals, primarily in urine and sweat. Since several of the minerals are stored in the body to cover any losses, an iron loss would not be noticed right away. But over many months or years, iron-deficiency anemia and osteoporosis could develop if the mineral store becomes drained.

Minerals in Food

Nearly all foods and beverages—even water—contain a mixture of minerals. As minerals originate from soil and water, foods like vegetables, fruits, and grains, and even products made from animals that eat plants and drink water, are great sources of minerals.

Some foods are better sources of minerals than others, because the amount of mineral available—able to be absorbed—from foods varies. For example, about 30 percent of the iron in red meat is able to be absorbed, as opposed to less than 10 percent of the iron in grain foods such as bread.

In summary, eating a wide variety of foods ensures sufficient intake of the minerals, just as it does with vitamins.

A List of the Minerals

Calcium

Function: Used for bone and tooth structure; muscle contraction; blood clotting; healthy nerve function.

Food Source: Milk products; green leafy vegetables, sardines with bones.

Chloride

Function: Works with sodium to maintain fluid balance; aids in digestion.

Food Source: Foods with salt (sodium chloride).

Magnesium

Function: Aids in normal nerve and muscle function; part of bone mineral structure.

Food Source: Green vegetables; beans; nuts; cocoa and chocolate products; whole grains.

Phosphorus

Function: Combines with calcium for healthy bone and tooth structure; used in energy metabolism; is part of every cell's genetic material.

Food Source: Meat; fish; poultry; milk products; beans.

Potassium

Function: Works with sodium to maintain fluid balance; helps control acid balance in the body.

Food Source: Whole foods—vegetables; fruits; meats; dairy products.

Sodium

Function: Vital for fluid balance and normal nervous system function.

Food Source: Salt; processed foods; soy sauce; other seasonings.

Chromium

Function: Needed for carbohydrate metabolism.

Food Source: Whole grains; vegetables; organ meats; brewer's yeast.

Copper

Function: Essential for blood cell and connective tissue formation.

Food Source: Whole grains; shell fish; organ meats; legumes.

Fluoride

Function: Makes tooth enamel more resistant to decay.

Food Source: Water containing fluorides; fish; tea.

Iodine

Function: Needed for thyroid hormone controlling the basal metabolism and weight gain.

Food Source: Milk products; whole-grains; iodized salt.

Iron

Function: Important for oxygen transport and energy metabolism.

Food Source: Red meat; poultry; fish; green leafy vegetables; whole grains; legumes.

Manganese

Function: Used in bone and connective tissue formation; carbohydrate and fat metabolism.

Food Source: Spinach; pumpkin; nuts; legumes; tea.

Molybdenum

Function: Needed for nitrogen metabolism.

Food Source: Unprocessed whole grains; vegetables.

Selenium

Function: With vitamin E it helps protect body tissue from oxidation and other aging processes.

Food Sources: Whole grains; meat; fish; poultry.

Zinc

Function: Used for wound healing; growth; appetite; sperm production.

Food Sources: Seafood; meats; nuts; legumes.

Vitamin and Mineral Supplements

Many individuals have already made the choice to use supplements, whether they need to or not. Supplements are taken for various reasons, including:

- To make up for poor eating habits
- As insurance against common illness
- To help combat stress at work and home

- To aid in weight loss or maintenance
- As prevention against long-term diseases like cancer, heart disease, and osteoporosis

Most of these reasons are not valid grounds for taking supplements. However, this does not mean that supplementation is useless and is not needed.

Valid Need of Supplementation

Here are several situations where a supplement may be beneficial, but not always necessary.

- **Alcohol Use**—It is well known that alcohol from beer, wine, and liquor interferes with vitamin and mineral metabolism. It also increases the loss of certain minerals in the urine, such as zinc.

- **Chronic Dieting**—Individuals who routinely consume less than 1,200-1,500 calories daily tend to miss the mark when meeting vitamin and mineral nutrient needs, since so little food is being consumed.

- **Food Allergies**—Certain types of foods may be the cause of allergic reactions in the body. Many foods, like wheat, fruit, or milk protein, have been found to be some of the top food allergies in the body.

- **Pregnancy**—Women who are pregnant have an increased need for many nutrients, all of which (except iron) can be met through a balanced diet. But in fact, all too often a supplement is recommended for the duration of the pregnancy.

- **Old Age**—Individuals over the age of 65 may have altered nutrient requirements that are not being met through the diet. This is because older individuals tend to consume less and have difficulty eating because of health problems or illnesses.

- **Medications**—Common drugs—antibiotics, analgesics, and oral contraceptives, for example—all interfere with vitamin and mineral utilization.

- **Vegetarian Diets**—When excluding meats, milk, eggs, and other animal products from the diet, alternative foods must replace the missing nutrients to meet the individual's needs.

Choosing a Supplement

Looking at the many aisles of supplements in a grocery store or health food store can be confusing and downright overwhelming. The following are four points for selecting safe and beneficial supplements:

- Select a supplement that contains a balance of 100-150 percent of the RDA for each vitamin and mineral
- Look for a one-per-day supplement and not one that has multiple dosages
- Avoid supplements labeled "high-potency" or "therapeutic," which tend to exceed the RDA and may be hazardous
- Choose a supplement based on its contents, not on a higher price

Supplementation Hazards

When the body has sufficient amounts of a particular vitamin or mineral, additional amounts do not enhance the function of that particular nutrient. Instead, the vitamin or mineral overload must be dealt with by the body. Either the excess is excreted in the urine (usually the water-soluble vitamins and some minerals) or stored in the body (usually fat-soluble vitamins and some minerals). In either case, one runs the risk of toxic side effects. The consequences of vitamin or mineral toxicity can be insignificant, but an excess of many vitamins and minerals can have dangerous consequences. It is also known that vitamin and mineral overdoses may mask medical disorders, interfere with the body's use of other nutrients, or precipitate a nutritional deficiency.

In summary, vitamin and mineral supplementation can be useful when needed and in small dosages. However, when vitamins and minerals are taken in excess, it poses a danger of toxicity in the body which can prove to be harmful.

CHAPTER 6
About Water and the Importance of It for the Body

Water is a very important nutrient for the body. In fact, the body can only survive a few days without water, while a deficiency of other nutrients may take weeks, months, and even years to develop.

Along with minerals, the body is able to maintain a proper balance and distribution of water. Approximately 50-75 percent of an individual's body weight is made up of water. The average body contains a total of 96 pints of water; 64 pints are found inside the body's cells, with the remainder outside the cells—in the blood, lymph fluid, and digestive juices.

Water and Body Fluids

In the body, water is the fluid in which all life processes take place. Each and every cell contains fluid of the exact composition that is best for that cell, known as intracellular fluid—the fluid within the cells, usually high in potassium and phosphate. The cell is bathed externally in what is known as interstitial fluid—the fluid between the cells, usually high in sodium and chloride. These particular fluids continually lose and restore their components, but the composition in each remains constant under normal circumstances. Whenever a disturbance occurs, the body quickly responds in order to keep the entire system of cells and fluids in a delicate balance of a state of homeostasis.

The purposes of water in the body are as follows:

- It carries nutrients and waste products throughout the body
- It participates in metabolic reactions
- It serves as the solvent for vitamins, minerals, glucose, amino acids, and many other small molecules

- It acts as a lubricant and a cushion around the joints, inside the eyes, and in the spinal cord; during pregnancy, the amniotic sac surrounds the fetus in the womb
- It aids in the regulation of body temperature
- It maintains blood volume

In order to support these functions and other important functions, the body is always maintaining a proper water balance.

Water Balance and Intake

Again, somewhere between 50-75 percent of an individual's body weight is made up of water. Since water makes up about three-fourths of the weight of lean tissue, and less than one-fourth of the weight of fat, an individual's body composition influences how much of the body's weight is water. It is known that the proportion of water is generally smaller in females, obese individuals, and the elderly, because of their smaller proportion of lean tissue. It is much higher in males, body builders, and athletes due to their larger proportion of lean tissue.

Due to the importance of water balance, the body attempts to restore homeostasis as promptly as possible, through adjusting both water intake and excretion as needed. The following are points on how the body is able to maintain proper water balance:

- **Water Sources**—The most obvious dietary sources of water is water itself and other beverages, but foods also contain water. Most vegetables and fruits are up to 90 percent water, while meats and cheeses are about 50 percent water. Fluid needs are best met by water, but milk and juices can account for part of the day's sources. Besides their high water content, these beverages deliver valuable nutrients to the body. However, alcoholic beverages and those containing caffeine (such as coffee, tea, and sodas) are not suitable substitutes for water. Both alcohol and caffeine act as diuretics, causing the body to lose about half the liquid consumed from the beverage. Also, during the breakdown of nutrients, the body produces water. On average, the body produces about 2.5 liters, or roughly 2.5 quarts of water from the processes of metabolism.

- **Water Recommendations**—A general requirement is difficult to establish, because water needs vary depending on diet, activity, environment temperature, and humidity. It is estimated that the average individual who expends 2,000 calories a day needs about 2-3 liters of water (about 7-11 cups). In addition to meeting the body's fluid needs, consuming plenty of water may protect the bladder against cancer and infections by diluting the urine and reducing its holding time. The risk of bladder cancer and infections is reduced when fluid intake is high.

- **Water Intake**—Thirst and satiety are the two main influences on water intake. This is likely because of the response to changes sensed by the mouth, hypothalamus, and nerves. For example, when the blood becomes concentrated—from lack or loss of water—the mouth becomes dry, and the hypothalamus initiates the drinking behavior. Receptors in the stomach send signals to stop the drinking behavior, as do receptors in the heart which monitor blood volume. Thirst drives an individual to seek water, but lags behind the body's need. Water deficiencies that develop slowly can switch on the drinking behavior in time to prevent serious dehydration. However, dehydration can easily develop with either water deprivation or excessive water loss. The signs of dehydration go from thirst to weakness, exhaustion, and delirium, and end in death if not addressed. On the other hand, water intoxication, which is rare, can occur with excessive water ingestion and kidney disorders that reduce urine output. The signs of water intoxication may include confusion and convulsions, and in some cases can result in death.

- **Water Losses**—The body excretes water every day through urine—enough to carry away the waste produced by a day's metabolic activities. Above this amount, excretion adjusts to balance intake. For example, if an individual drinks more water, the kidneys excrete more urine, and the urine becomes more diluted. Besides urine, water is lost from the lungs as vapor, from the skin as sweat, and some is lost in feces. The amount lost from each of these sources varies depending on activity, environment temperature, and humidity. But on average, the daily loss totals about 2.5 liters for most individuals.

In summary, water makes up about 75 percent of the body's weight, and assists with the transport of nutrients and waste products throughout the body. It also participates in chemical reactions, acts as a solvent, serves as a shock absorber, and regulates body temperature. In order to maintain water balance, consumption from liquids, foods, and metabolism must equal losses from the kidneys, lungs, skin, and feces.

Blood Volume and Blood Pressure

Water maintains the blood volume in the body, which in turn influences blood pressure. The kidneys are essential to the regulation of blood volume and blood pressure. They continually reabsorb needed substances and water and excrete waste with some water in the urine. Also, the kidneys carefully adjust the volume and the consistency of the urine to accommodate changes in the body, including variations in the day's food and fluid consumption. The following are other functions that take place in the body which assist in keeping the blood volume and blood pressure working optimally:

- **ADH and Water Retention**—When blood volume or blood pressure falls too low, or when the extracellular fluid becomes too concentrated, the hypothalamus signals the pituitary gland to release what is known as Antidiuretic Hormone, or ADH for short. The ADH is a water-conserving hormone that stimulates the kidneys to reabsorb water. As a result, the more water the body needs, the less the kidneys will excrete. (**Side Note:** When these events take place in the body, it triggers thirst. Drinking water will raise the blood volume and dilute the concentration of fluids, thus helping to restore homeostasis.)

- **Renin and Sodium Retention**—The cells in the kidneys respond to low blood pressure by releasing an enzyme known as renin. Through a series of complex events, renin causes the kidneys to reabsorb sodium. When sodium is reabsorbed, it is always accompanied by water retention, which helps to restore blood volume and blood pressure.

- **Angiotensin and Blood Vessel Constriction**—Not only is renin an enzyme from the kidneys, but it activates angiotensin. Angiotensin is a hormone involved in blood pressure regulation, and is a precursor protein known as angiotensinogen. (**Side Note**: Angiotensin is a very strong vasoconstrictor—a substance that constricts or narrows the diameters of blood vessels, thereby raising the blood pressure in the body.)

- **Aldosterone and Sodium Retention**—The Aldosterone signals the kidneys to retain more sodium and thus water, because when sodium moves, fluids follow. Once more, the effect is that when more water is needed, less is excreted. (**Side Note**: Angiotensin intercedes in the release of the hormone Aldosterone from the adrenal glands.)

In summary, all of these functions clarify why high-sodium diets aggravate conditions such as hypertension or edema. Excessive amounts of sodium cause water retention and an accompanying rise in blood pressure and/or swelling in the interstitial spaces. Also, these functions are able to maintain water balance only if an individual's intake of water is high enough.

Fluid and Electrolyte Balance

Maintaining the balance of the body fluids inside and outside the cells is critical to the life of the cells. If too much water were to enter the cells, it might rupture them; if too much water leaves, they would collapse. In order to keep a balance of water movement inside and outside the cells, the major minerals play a role in controlling the direction of the water movement.

A few electrolytes (sodium and chloride) reside primarily outside the cells, while others (potassium, magnesium, phosphate, and sulfate) are predominantly inside the cells. It is known that cell membranes are selectively permeable, meaning that they allow the passage of some molecules, but not of others. When electrolytes move across the membrane, water follows.

The amount of varying minerals in the body must remain nearly constant, in order to regulate the fluid and electrolyte balance. This regulation starts in two main sites: the GI tract and the kidneys.

The GI tract is known to continuously deliver minerals to the stomach and small intestine in the digestive juices and bile it secretes. It then reabsorbs these minerals and those from foods in the large intestine when needed; thereby providing ample opportunity for the regulation of electrolyte balance.

The kidneys control the body's water balance by way of the hormone ADH. In order to regulate the electrolyte balance, the kidneys depend on the adrenal glands, which send out messages via the hormone Aldosterone. When the body's sodium level is low, Aldosterone stimulates sodium reabsorption from the kidneys. While sodium is reabsorbed, potassium is excreted accordingly.

Fluid and Electrolyte Imbalance

Generally, the body defends itself successfully against fluid and electrolyte imbalances, but in certain situations its ability to compensate and correct itself may not occur. For example, vomiting, diarrhea, heavy sweating, burns, and wounds may incur such a great fluid and electrolyte loss or imbalance at to precipitate a medical crisis.

Sodium and chloride are the two electrolytes that are most easily lost in the body. They are first lost by sweating, bleeding, or excretion. However, if fluids are lost by vomiting or diarrhea, sodium is lost indiscriminately. In many cases, individuals are able to replace the fluids and electrolytes lost in sweat or in a temporary bout of diarrhea by drinking plain cool water and eating whole foods such as fruits, vegetables, and grains. Other cases demand rapid replacement of lost fluids and electrolytes, such as when diarrhea threatens a malnourished child, an elderly person, or someone suffering from an eating disorder. In such cases, hospitalization is required to restore balance to the fluids and electrolytes in the body.

Acid-Base Balance

The acidity of the body's fluids is determined by the concentration of hydrogen ions. A high concentration of hydrogen ions would be very acidic. The body uses its ions not only to help maintain fluid and electrolyte balance, but to regulate the acidity of pH of its fluids. Ordinary energy metabolism generates hydrogen ions, as well as other acids that must be neutralized.

The three systems known to defend the body against fluctuations in pH are buffers in the blood, respiration in the lungs, and excretion in the kidneys. A summary of each of these systems follows:

- **Regulation by the Buffers**—Buffers known as bicarbonate (a base) and carbonic (an acid) in the body fluids, as well as proteins, protect the body against changes in acidity. Bicarbonate and carbonic acid are substances that are able to neutralize acids or bases. These buffer systems serve as the first line of defense against changes in the fluids' acid-base balance.

- **Regulation by the Lungs**—Respiration supplies another defense. Carbon dioxide, which is formed all the time during cellular metabolism, forms carbonic acid in the blood, therefore pushing the balance toward acid. However, if too much acid builds up, the respiration rate speeds up. This hyperventilation increases the amount of carbon dioxide exhaled, thus lowering the carbonic acid concentration and restoring homeostasis. On the other hand, if base builds up, the respiration rate slows and carbon dioxide is retained and forms more carbonic acid. As a result, homeostasis is restored.

- **Regulation by the Kidneys**—The kidneys play a key role in maintaining long-term control of acid-base balance. It does this by selecting which ions to retain and to excrete. The kidneys are adjusting the body's acid-base balance nearly constantly. The body's total acid load remains constant; urine's acidity fluctuates in order to accommodate that balance.

In summary, electrolytes in fluids help to distribute the fluids inside and outside the cells, making the appropriate water balance and acid-base balance in order to support all the body's processes. Excessive loss of fluids and electrolytes upset these balances, and the kidneys play a vital role in restoring homeostasis.

Overview of Water Sources

A number of health-seeking individuals are turning to the wide array of bottled waters available as their main source of water for consumption. The following are descriptions of some of the common waters on the market today:

- **Drinking Water**—Noncarbonated water that is typically used as an alternative to tap water. The source of drinking water is variable and may be a municipal water supply, not necessarily a well or spring.

- **Sparkling Water**—Carbon dioxide is introduced to make it bubbly. Natural sparkling water has enough carbon dioxide occurring naturally in the water that it has a bubbly fizz already.

- **Distilled Water**—Has been vaporized and condensed, and thus contains no minerals. It may contain microorganisms or organics sloughed off from ion-exchange purifiers.

- **Spring Water**—Flows out of the earth, is bottled near its source, and is not altered by adding anything or by taking away the minerals or carbonation present.

- **Mineral Water**—Contains a variety of minerals—primarily calcium, magnesium, and sodium—naturally present in the water source. Mineral content varies depending on the source, but nearly all waters, with the exception of distilled and purified water, contain some minerals.

- **Seltzer Water**—Usually plain old tap water with added fizz, but no added minerals. Many seltzers have added sweeteners like corn syrup or sucrose. Unlike other bottled waters, seltzers are not necessarily calorie-free.

- **Club Soda**—Artificially carbonated tap water with added minerals and salts.

Fluid Replacement Guide

Whether an individual is in the office at work or pushing through a workout at the gym, lost body fluids mean lagging performance. Constantly hectic schedules, missed meals, exercise, traveling, weather changes, and long work days interfere with replenishing lost fluid. The following are simple guidelines of what, when, and how much to drink, along with tips on how to minimize water loss and optimize water replenishment.

- **Start with 8-16 ounces of water**—Upon waking up in the morning, the body is already facing a water deficit. Instead of starting the day with a dehydrating cup of coffee or tea, drink a good cup or two of water before or along with breakfast.

- **Keep fluids readily accessible**—To keep up with fluid needs, keep water or other healthy beverages close at hand. Have bottled water in the car during the commute, by your desk at work, or on the kitchen counter at home.

- **Take planned water breaks**—Whether at home, at work, or out running errands, take time to drink some water at least every 30-45 minutes. This will help maintain hydration in the body.

- **Be aware of the signs of dehydration**—Think about consuming fluids when the signs of dehydration—dryness of the eyes, nose, or mouth—start to become evident. These symptoms normally occur when breathing dry air, traveling, working outside in the heat, or experiencing a change in climate.

- **Avoid dehydrating food and drink**—Salty foods temporarily increase the body's need for fluid, and the body works to maintain a constant salt concentration in the blood and tissues. Extra salt needs to be diluted with additional water, and will eventually be excreted as urine by the kidneys, whose job is to regulate sodium levels in the body. Beverages containing caffeine—like coffee, teas, and some sodas—and alcoholic beverages change fluid needs. These beverages all act like diuretics, increasing water loss in the body.

- **Don't skip meals**—When a meal is missed, the body is robbed not only of nutrients, but of water. Much of the daily fluid consumption comes during meals. Foods as well as beverages supply water.

- **Hydrate well before, during, and after air travel**—Try to consume about 8-16 ounces of water before a flight. This hydration helps minimize the dehydrating effects of air travel. Hold on to beverage cups on long flights and ask for refills, or bring a bottle of water to drink during the flight.

- **Be aware of weather changes**—A rise in the outside heat means the body will adjust to the new temperature by sweating, to cool off the skin. Feeling thirsty can be delayed when it is hot and fluid loss is more rapid. Drink more fluids in warmer weather, higher humidity, and higher altitudes, because these cause greater water loss in the body.

- **Hydrate well before, during, and after exercise**—During exercise—whatever the type—the body generates heat. Dissipating this heat requires fluid evaporation from the skin (sweating), which cools the body. In an effort to stay cool, the body loses valuable water. As a result, the blood thickens, the heart rate goes up, and body temperature starts to climb. If water loss continues, symptoms of dehydration will become prominent and should be treated. Since dehydration can threaten not only performance but the individual's life as well, action needs to be taken before, during, and after exercise, to ensure that adequate fluids are available to the body. During exercise, experiment with drinking at regular intervals. Developing the best fluid replacement plan during exercise will even improve performance.

In summary, it is vitally important to keep the body well hydrated at all times. Fluids or water play an important part in all the body's functions, and help to maintain a state of homeostasis as well. Do you drink enough water?

PART 2
Life Cycle Nutrition

CHAPTER 7
Pregnancy and Lactation

A whole new life begins at conception. Organ systems start to rapidly develop, and nutrition plays a significant supportive role in this new life.

Placenta Development

In the early days of pregnancy, what is known as the placenta develops within the uterus. Two other structures also form:

- **Amniotic Sac**—A fluid-filled, balloon-like structure that houses the developing fetus

- **Umbilical Cord**—A ropelike structure containing fetal blood vessels that extends through the fetus's belly button to the placenta

The placenta develops as an interweaving of fetal and maternal blood vessels embedded in the uterine wall. The maternal blood transfers oxygen and nutrients to the fetus's blood and picks up fetal waste products. Therefore, by exchanging oxygen, nutrients, and waste products, the placenta performs the respiratory, absorptive, and excretory functions which the fetus's lungs, digestive system, and kidneys will provide once the fetus is fully developed, after birth.

The placenta is a resourceful, metabolically active organ which uses energy and nutrients to support its work. Like a gland, it produces an array of hormones that maintain the pregnancy and prepare the mother's breast for lactation (making milk). A healthy placenta is essential for the developing fetus to grow and reach its full potential.

Overview of Fetal Growth and Development

Weeks 1-2

Fertilization is the joining of the sperm and the egg in the fallopian tube to form a unique human life. Forty-six chromosomes provide the blueprint for the embryo's physical characteristics.

Week 3

At this point, the developing embryo is looking for a spot to implant in the uterus. Early formation of the central nervous system, backbone, and spinal column has begun. The gastrointestinal system has also begun to develop, with the kidneys, liver, and intestines forming. The heart has begun to form.

Week 4

Hormones produced by the embryo stop the mother's menstrual cycle.

Week 5

The embryo's tiny heart begins to beat by day twenty-one. The brain has developed into five areas and some cranial nerves are visible. Arm and leg buds are visible, and the formation of the eyes, lips, and nose has begun. The spinal cord grows faster than the rest of the body, giving a tail-like appearance which disappears as the embryo continues to grow. The placenta begins to provide nourishment for the embryo.

Weeks 6-7

Major organs have all begun to form. The embryo has developed its own blood type, unique from the mother's. Hair follicles and nipples form, and knees and elbows are visible. Facial features are also observable. The eyes have a retina and lens. The major muscle system is developed and the embryo is able to move.

Week 8

The embryo is reactive to its environment inside the amniotic sac where it swims and moves. Hands and feet can be seen. At the end of week 8, the embryonic period is over and the fetal stage begins.

Weeks 9-12

The heart is almost completely developed. Most major organs and tissues have developed, and red blood cells are now produced in the liver. The face is well formed and the eyes are almost fully developed. The eyelids will close and not reopen until the 28th week. Arms, hands, fingers, legs, feet, and toes are fully formed. Nails and earlobes start to form, and tooth buds develop in the gums. Fetus can make a fist with its full hand and fingers. Testosterone (male sex hormone) is produced by the testes in a male fetus.

Weeks 13-16

The brain is fully developed, and the fetus can suck, swallow, and make irregular breathing sounds. The fetus can feel pain and the fetal skin is almost transparent. Muscles tissue is lengthening and bones are becoming harder. Liver and organs produce appropriate fluids. Eyebrows and eyelashes appear, and the fetus makes active movements, including kicks and even somersaults.

Weeks 17-20

Usually around this time the finger and toenails appear. Lanugo, a fine hair, now covers the entire body, and the fetus can hear and recognize the mother's voice. Sex organs are visible on ultrasound devices.

Weeks 21-24

A protective waxy substance known as vernix covers the skin. By birth, most of the vernix will be gone, but any that is left is quickly absorbed. The fetus has startle reflex. Footprints and fingerprints are forming. The fetus practices breathing by inhaling amniotic fluid into its developing lungs.

Weeks 25-28

Rapid brain development occurs during this period, and the nervous system is able to control some bodily functions. The eyelids now open and close. At 25 weeks, there is a 60 percent chance of survival if born. The fetus is considered legally viable at 28 weeks, and there is a 90 percent chance of survival if born at that point.

Weeks 29-32

There is a rapid increase in the amount of body fat the fetus has. Rhythmic breathing occurs, but the lungs are not yet mature. The fetus sleeps 90-95 percent of the day. At this point, the survival rate is above 95 percent if the baby is born.

Weeks 33-40

The fetus is considered full-term. Lanugo is gone except on upper arms and shoulders. Hair on the baby's head is now coarser and thicker. The lungs are mature. The average weight of the baby at this point is seven and a half pounds. At birth, the placenta detaches from the uterus and the umbilical cord will be cut as the baby takes the first breaths of air. Breathing will trigger changes in the heart and bypass arteries, forcing all blood to travel through the lungs.

Nutrition During Pregnancy

Pregnancy introduces a host of physiological and emotional changes in a woman. Advice seems to pour in from all sources: one's obstetrician, well-meaning friends and family members, and colleagues at work. Even perfect strangers have been known to put in their two cents when it comes to commenting on a pregnant woman's health.

In the face of often-contradictory advice—especially in regard to one's diet—it may be hard for a mom-to-be to achieve a comfortable and healthy balance. Eating a healthy diet is one of the most vital things any pregnant woman can do to enhance her body's health as well as the health of the growing fetus. It is important to consume a healthy and balanced diet now and after the birth of the baby.

Weight Gain

Gaining the right amount of weight when you are pregnant is important. It is one measure of the healthy growth of your baby, especially after the first three months of pregnancy. Your weight gain also affects your baby's birth weight. Studies have shown that babies with birth weights in the range of 5.5 to 9 pounds tend to be healthier. The number of pounds you should gain while you are pregnant depends on your weight before pregnancy and your height.

Recommended Total Weight Gain

- Women who are underweight for height—28-40 lbs.

- Women who are normal weight for height—25-35 lbs.

- Women who are overweight for height—15-25 lbs.

Studies show that shorter women should gain near the lower end of the range; black women and very young women should gain close to the upper end of the range. The recommended gain for women who are carrying twins is 35-45 pounds. (**Side Note:** Pregnancy is not the time to diet to lose weight. Gaining too little weight during pregnancy may produce a baby too small at birth. Gaining too much weight during pregnancy can cause problems such as high blood pressure, diabetes, and a difficult delivery. It can also result in very large babies [more than 9 pounds], who are more likely to have health problems than smaller babies.)

Rate of Weight Gain

During your first 3 months of pregnancy, you will usually gain 2-4 pounds. When your baby begins to grow fast, you gain roughly a pound per week (more if you are underweight, less if you are overweight). Small differences in this rate are not important.

Mild swelling during the last 3 months of pregnancy is normal. If your legs, ankles, or feet become puffy, put your feet on a stool or chair for a while. A large, sudden weight gain accompanied by swelling of your hands and face is not normal and needs medical attention quickly.

Recommended Calorie Levels

To meet your extra food needs for a healthy weight gain, you need to add an average of 300 extra calories per day to your diet after the first 3 months of pregnancy. (**Side Note**: If you exercise during pregnancy, you may need to add more than 300 calories per day.)

Add these extra calories with an additional serving of milk, low-fat cheese, lean meats, poultry, fish, leafy and dark green vegetables, dried beans and peas, fruits, whole grains, and enriched breads and cereals.

Don't eat lots of cookies, candies, cakes, chips, soft drinks, and fats, such as butter, margarine, gravy, fried foods, salad dressings, and mayonnaise. These high-calorie foods provide very little nourishment for you and the developing fetus.

Daily Food Guide for Pregnant Women

During pregnancy, especially the first three months or so, the body's hormones are fluctuating. So is the blood sugar level, which can lead to fatigue, queasiness, and nausea. This is known as morning sickness. For the most part, it can be controlled by diet, by frequently consuming a balance of carbohydrates and low-fat proteins throughout the day.

The goal is to eat small meals every 2-3 hours to prevent morning sickness, rather than trying to treat it after it hits by eating. Be aware of how your body is feeling and eat accordingly, in order to help it operate efficiently while pregnant.

Sample Day Meal Plan

Breakfast:
2 slices whole grain toast
2 Tbsp. peanut butter and 1 Tbsp. honey
1 cup low-fat milk
Orange slices

Midmorning Snack:
5 whole grain crackers
1 oz. sliced cheese

Lunch:
Roast beef and cheese sandwich (2 slices whole wheat bread, 1 Tbsp. low-fat mayo, lettuce, tomato, 2 oz. roast beef, 1 oz. cheese)
½ cup carrot sticks
1 cup low-fat milk

Midday Snack:
½ cup trail mix (a combination of peanuts, almonds, sunflower

seeds, pumpkin seeds, and raisins)

Dinner:
3 oz. steak
1 cup wild rice
½ cup steamed broccoli
1 whole wheat roll

Night Snack:
1 cup low-fat yogurt with ½ cup granola

Other Nutrient Needs

The body's needs for almost all nutrients (vitamins and minerals) are greater when you are pregnant. Nutrients are important in your own body's growth, your baby's, and later for breast-feeding. The amount of iron and folate in your diet is important, so eat foods containing these nutrients often.

- **Iron**—This mineral carries oxygen to your baby. You need more iron than you normally do for the baby, and it is hard to get enough from foods alone. Your doctor will probably recommend an iron supplement while you are pregnant. Taking an iron supplement between meals or at bedtime on an empty stomach helps to increase its absorption. It is also important to eat iron-rich foods daily.

- **Folate or Folic Acid**—This B vitamin helps your body make red blood cells and genes. The amount of folate you need more than doubles when you are pregnant. Eating various foods that contain folate is the best way to get enough.

The following are food sources of iron and folate:

Iron Sources:

- Lean meat, poultry, fish, organ meats (such as liver)
- Dried beans and peas (such as lima, navy, kidney, and pinto beans, and split green and black-eyed peas)

- Dark-green vegetables (such as collard greens, turnip greens, mustard greens, spinach, and broccoli)
- Whole-grain and enriched breads and cereals (such as whole-wheat bread, pumpernickel bread, bran muffin, oatmeal, fortified ready-to-eat cereals)

Folate Sources:

- Liver
- Dried beans and peas (such as black-eyed peas; red, kidney, or white beans; butter beans; lentils)
- Dark-green leafy vegetables (such as spinach, broccoli, turnip greens, mustard greens, collards, romaine lettuce)
- Whole-grain breads and cereals, cereals fortified with folic acid (check the label)
- Fruit (such as oranges and orange juice, grapefruit, bananas, cantaloupe, and tomatoes and tomato juice)

(**Side Note:** The iron in meat, fish, and poultry is more readily absorbed by the body than the iron in plant foods. To increase iron absorption, eat plant foods with meat or with foods that contain vitamin C. Some good sources of vitamin C are oranges, grapefruits, tangerines, strawberries, potatoes, and bell peppers.)

Vitamin and Mineral Supplements

Although vitamin and mineral supplements are common, extra servings of healthy foods are the best sources for most women. Also, supplements may not contain all the essential nutrients supplied by healthy foods, which are less likely to cause unhealthy nutrient interactions.

Taking too many vitamin or mineral supplements can harm the fetus. More than 150 percent of the Recommended Dietary Allowance (RDA) shown on the label is considered too much. Most damage occurs during the first 3 months, when you may not know you are pregnant. However, you may need a multivitamin and mineral supplement if these conditions apply to you:

- Poor diet that is lacking in any of the basic food groups

- Pregnant with more than one baby
- Smoke, drink alcohol, or use drugs

Basic Supplementation During Pregnancy

Nutrient: Calcium

Use: Baby's bone development; mother's bone strength; prevents muscle cramps.

Sources: Dairy products; dark vegetables; salmon; dried beans.

Nutrient: Copper

Use: Preventing anemia; forming baby's bone and nerve fibers.

Sources: Dried beans; nuts; seeds; raisins; whole grains.

Nutrient: Cyanocobalamin (B-12)

Use: Preventing anemia.

Sources: Dairy products; meats; eggs.

Nutrient: Vitamin C

Use: Preventing anemia; building strong bones and teeth.

Sources: Citrus; broccoli; mangoes; red peppers; strawberries.

Nutrient: Folic Acid

Use: Helps in preventing neural tube defects; red blood cell and cell turnover; helps to utilize proteins.

Sources: Dark vegetables; oranges; dried beans; whole; grains.

Nutrient: Iron

Use: Preventing anemia; helps baby's weight gain; prevents premature delivery.

Sources: Meats; dried fruit; whole grains; green vegetables.
Nutrient: Magnesium

Use: Bone and tissue building; nerve transmissions; immune function.

Sources: Whole grains; beans; fish; dark vegetables.

Nutrient: Pyridoxine (B-6)

Use: Helps in utilizing proteins; aids in cell turnover and production.

Sources: Whole grains; eggs; meat; dried beans; nuts; bananas; avocados.

Nutrient: Riboflavin

Use: Preventing anemia; building baby's cells and tissues; helps to utilize energy nutrients.

Sources: Dairy products; eggs; whole grains; dark meats.
Nutrient: Selenium

Use: Protects body from free radicals; aids in reducing cancer risk.

Sources: Brazil nuts; whole grains; fish; meat.

Nutrient: Zinc

Use: Cell division; aids proper growth; prevents premature births; achieves muscle strength; aids in endurance and healing.

Sources: Meats; fish; whole grains; dried beans; nuts; beets; carrots; cabbage.

Supplement May Be Needed in Special Circumstances

- **Vitamin B12**—Supplements may be needed if you are a vegetarian and eat no animal foods.
- **Vitamin D**—Supplements may be needed to help in proper bone development.
- **Calcium**—Supplements may be needed if you are under age 25, especially if you do not consume enough foods that contain calcium. (**Side Note**: take calcium supplements at mealtimes so they do not inhibit the absorption of iron supplements. Plus it is best to take a magnesium supplement along with the calcium supplement to aid in the absorption of the calcium supplement in the body.)
- **Zinc**—Supplements may be needed in the DNA and RNA synthesis and for protein synthesis for proper cell development.

Making Nutrition Part of Your Life During Pregnancy

Choose foods that you like, and do not try to force yourself to eat foods that you dislike. Be realistic and plan meals that will fit your lifestyle. If you are always rushing in the morning, try to plan some simple but nourishing meals that can be eaten in a hurry. A bran muffin, a glass of milk, and an orange are one suggestion.

It is also a good idea to plan ahead so you don't just grab what's there when you are hungry. Pregnancy is not the time to snack on a bag of chips and a soft drink. Try some cheese, crackers, and fruit for a quick snack when away from home.

The following breakfast, lunch, dinner, and snack samples are very nutritious and not difficult or time-consuming to prepare.

Breakfast Ideas

The following are some breakfast ideas that are very nutritious:

- Berry protein drink with whole grain bagel

- Waffles with honey
  Egg
  Orange slices

- Oatmeal with granola, nuts and raisins
  Milk

- Toast with jelly
  Potatoes
  Eggs

- French toast with honey
  Fresh fruit salad

- Yogurt with granola and nuts
  Whole grain bagel

- Toast with peanut butter and jelly
  Milk

Lunch Ideas
The following are some lunch ideas that are very nutritious:

- Pizza
  Tossed salad with dressing

- Chicken sandwich
  Carrot sticks
  Milk

- Garden salad with chicken and dressing
  Whole grain roll

- Pasta
  Tossed salad with dressing
  Whole grain roll

- Turkey and cheese sandwich
  Orange slices

- Bean burritos
  Tortilla chips

- Roast beef and cheese sandwich
  Apple slices

- Peanut butter and jelly sandwich
  Carrot sticks
  Milk

Dinner Ideas

The following are some dinner ideas that are very nutritious:

- Cube steak
  Tater tots
  Tossed salad with dressing
  Steamed carrots

- Grilled steak
  Baked potato with sour cream
  Tossed salad with dressing
  Steamed broccoli

- Lasagna
  Tossed salad with dressing
  Whole grain roll

- Pizza
  Tossed salad with low-fat dressing

- Grilled chicken
  Couscous
  Tossed salad with dressing
  Steamed peas

- Fettuccine Alfredo

Tossed salad with dressing
Whole grain roll

- Chicken fajitas
  Fresh fruit salad

Snack Ideas

The following are some snack ideas that are very nutritious:

- Apple and a cheese stick

- Whole grain bagel with cream cheese

- Trail mix and dried fruit

- Protein drinks/smoothies

- Yogurt with granola and nuts

- Cottage cheese with pineapple

- Graham crackers with 2 Tbsp. of peanut butter

- 2 oz. lean meat with whole grain crackers

In summary, energy and nutrient needs during pregnancy are higher and can be met through eating a healthy and balanced diet.

Practices Incompatible with Pregnancy
Alcohol

We know that drinking alcoholic beverages can be dangerous to unborn babies, yet many women continue to drink wine, beer, or liquor during pregnancy.

More than 50 percent of the babies born to alcoholic mothers have what is known as Fetal Alcohol Syndrome (FAS). These infants have birth defects, mental retardation, and a reduced growth rate. Even if alcohol intake does not cause full-blown FAS, it is associated with miscarriage, low birth weight, and learning disorders.

No safe level of alcohol consumption has been established for pregnant women. Some studies show that as few as one or two drinks per day may be harmful to the developing fetus. Both the Food and Drug Administration (FDA) and the U.S. Surgeon General have recommended that pregnant women avoid drinking any alcohol during pregnancy. Damage may occur during the first 3 months before a woman knows she is pregnant. Avoid alcohol if you are even considering pregnancy.

Caffeine

Caffeine is a stimulant found in coffee, tea, colas, other soft drinks, chocolate, cocoa, and some drugs. Whether a pregnant woman should avoid caffeine is still open to question.

Pregnant women who choose to consume foods and drinks containing caffeine should do so in moderation. Use all drugs only on the advice of your doctor.

Smoking

Smoking cigarettes at any time poses harmful effects, and during pregnancy it is dramatically magnified. Smoking restricts the blood flow to the growing fetus, and so limits oxygen and nutrient delivery and waste removal. Also, smokers tend to consume less nutritious foods during pregnancy than do non-smokers, which further impairs fetal development. A more detailed list of complications associated with smoking during pregnancy is as follows:

- Fetal growth retardation
- Low birth weight
- Complications at birth
- Miss-location of the placenta
- Premature separation of the placenta
- Vaginal bleeding
- Spontaneous abortion
- Fetal death
- Sudden Infant Death Syndrome (SIDS)
- Middle ear disease
- Cardiac and respiratory disease

Medicinal Drugs

All drugs other than alcohol can also cause complications during pregnancy, problems in labor, and a number of serious birth defects. When pregnant, medicinal drugs should not be taken without consulting a doctor.

Herbal Supplements

Similarly, when pregnant it is important to seek out the advice of a doctor before continuing the use of herbal supplements. Most herbal supplements are safe, but some can be harmful.

Weight Loss and/or Dieting

Weight loss or dieting, even for short periods during pregnancy, is not healthy and is hazardous to the fetus. Regardless of pregnancy weight, it is important to never intentionally lose weight or go on a diet.

In summary, proper nutrition and abstinence from smoking, alcohol, and other drugs will help increase the likelihood of a safe and healthy pregnancy overall.

Common Problems During Pregnancy
Nausea or Vomiting

Nausea (morning sickness) can occur at any time of the day, but it is often most troublesome when you get up in the morning. The problem is usually mild, and it often goes away after the first 3 months of pregnancy. You can stop or reduce your nausea and vomiting if you take these precautions:

- Eat a few crackers, a handful of dry cereal, or a piece of dry toast or bread before you get out of bed in the morning. Put these within easy reach the night before.
- Get up slowly in the morning. Avoid sudden movements.
- Eat five or six small meals a day. Never go for long periods without food. Try not to get hungry.
- Drink fluids, including soups, between meals rather than with them.
- Drink a small amount of apple juice, grape juice, or a carbonated beverage if you feel nauseated between meals.

- Avoid greasy fried foods and other foods that upset your stomach, such as highly seasoned foods.
- Open windows or use the exhaust fan to get rid of odors when you cook.
- Have plenty of fresh air in the room while you are sleeping.

Constipation

During pregnancy, your digestive system relaxes so that your body can absorb more nutrients. This relaxation can cause constipation. During your last 3 months of pregnancy, your uterus will apply pressure to the large intestine, aggravating the problem. These suggestions may help:

- Eat more raw fruits and vegetables (including the skins), dried fruits, stewed prunes or apricots, and prune juice.
- Eat whole grain products, such as oatmeal or brown rice, and whole wheat breads. Sprinkle wheat germ or bran on cereal, or have a bran muffin.
- Eat more dried beans and peas.
- Drink more liquids, including water, milk, fruit juices, and soups.
- Eat meals at regular times.
- Exercise regularly if possible.

Heartburn

Especially in late pregnancy, your uterus will push up on your stomach. After you eat, swallowed food can be forced back up. This causes a burning feeling called heartburn. Eating five to six small meals a day, rather than two or three large ones, often relieves this discomfort. Avoid fatty, fried, and spicy foods.

Hemorrhoids

Some women already have hemorrhoids, and others develop them during the last 3 months of pregnancy. The reason is the weight of the baby. The suggestions for relieving constipation also help with hemorrhoids.

Cravings

Some women crave nonfood items, such as clay, dirt, or starch when they are pregnant. Try not to eat these because they do not provide nutrients that you and your baby need. They may also block the nutrients from foods that you do eat.

In summary, the nausea, constipation, heartburn, and hemorrhoids that sometimes accompany pregnancy can usually be alleviated with a few simple strategies. Food cravings do not typically reflect physiological needs and are best satisfied with a balanced meal or snack.

Nutrition During Lactation

During pregnancy, the breasts begin to prepare for being the main source of nourishment for the newborn infant. Breast-feeding offers many health benefits to both mother and infant. Still, there are those who consider an alternative, such as infant formula, in place of breast milk.

Lactation

Lactation naturally follows pregnancy, and the mammary glands—the glands of the female breast—secrete milk for this purpose. The mammary glands develop during puberty but remain fairly inactive until pregnancy. During pregnancy, hormones promote the growth and branching of the duct system in the breasts and the development of the milk-producing cells.

At this point, the hormones prolactin and oxytocin finely coordinate lactation. As the infant nurses, it stimulates the release of these hormones, which signal the mammary glands to supply milk. Prolactin concentrations remain high and milk production continues as long as the infant is nursing.

Oxytocin causes the mammary glands to eject milk into the ducts, which is known as the let-down reflex. It is normal to be able to feel this reflex as a contraction of the breast, flowed by the flow of milk and the release of pressure. (**Side Note:** By relaxing and eating well, the nursing mother promotes easy let-down of milk and greatly enhances the chances of successful lactation.)

Breast-feeding

It has been established that lactation is an automatic physiological process, which naturally occurs in the body during a pregnancy. Breast-feeding, on the other hand, is a learned behavior that not all mothers care to do.

Most healthy mothers who choose to breast-feed can do so with little preparation; physical obstacles to breast-feeding are rare. Successful breast-feeding requires adequate nutrition and proper rest. This, in addition to the support of all who care, will help to enhance the well-being of mother and infant.

There are many benefits to breast-feeding. Even if a mother is only able to do it for a short time, the infant's immune system can benefit from breast milk. Here are many other benefits of breast milk for the infant and mother:

Benefits for the Infant:

- Breast milk is the most complete form of nutrition for infants. A mother's milk has just the right amount of fat, sugar, water, and protein that is needed for an infant's growth and development. Most infants find it easier to digest breast milk than they do formula.
- As a result, breast-fed infants grow exactly the way they should. They tend to gain less unnecessary weight and tend to be leaner. This may result in being less overweight later in life.
- Premature infants do better when breast-fed compared to premature infants who are fed formula.
- Breast-fed infants score slightly higher on IQ tests, especially infants who were born prematurely.
- Infants who are breast-fed are not sick as often and have fewer doctors' visits.
- Breast milk has agents (called antibodies) in it to help protect infants from bacteria and viruses.

Benefits for the Mother:

- Nursing uses up extra calories, making it easier to lose the pounds of pregnancy. It also helps the uterus to get back to its original size, and lessens any bleeding a woman may have after giving birth.

- Breast-feeding, especially exclusive breast-feeding (no supplementing with formula), delays the return of normal ovulation and menstrual cycles. (However, you should still talk with your doctor or nurse about birth control choices.)
- Breast-feeding lowers the risk of breast and ovarian cancers, and possibly the risk of hip fractures and osteoporosis after menopause.
- Breast-feeding makes your life easier. It saves time and money. You do not have to purchase, measure, and mix formula. There are no bottles to warm in the middle of the night!
- A mother can give her infant immediate satisfaction by providing her breast milk when her infant is hungry.
- Breast-feeding requires a mother to take some quiet relaxed time for herself and her infant.
- Breast-feeding can help a mother to bond with her infant. Physical contact is important to newborns and can help them feel more secure, warm and comforted.
- Breast-feeding mothers may have increased self-confidence and feelings of closeness with their infants.

Mother's Nutrient Needs

When the mother chooses to breast-feed, her infant will continue to get nutrient-dense foods throughout lactation. A balanced healthy diet is needed to support the stamina, patience, and self-confidence that nursing the demands of an infant.

The following are helpful points to keep in mind when breast-feeding:

- **Nutrient Intake and Exercise**—It is estimated that a nursing mother produces about 25 ounces of milk per day, depending on the infant's demand for milk. In order to produce an adequate supply of milk, it is important to increase nutrient intake by almost 650 calories per day (above meeting normal nutrient needs) for the first six months of lactation. It is advised that about 500 extra calories per day be consumed, and that the fat reserves accumulated during pregnancy provide the remaining 150 calories. When breast-feeding, the nutrient intake range is from 2,500-3,300 calories per day, depending on physical activity. After giving birth, many women are anxious to lose the extra body fat they accumulated during pregnancy. There are differences of opinion on whether or not breast-feeding aids in postpartum weight loss. It has been noted that most women lose one to two pounds per month during the first four to six months of lactation; some may lose more, some less. Women who exercise before, during and after pregnancy seem to maintain a gradual weight loss and end up at their pre-pregnancy weight. (**Side Note**: Exercise is completely compatible with breast-feeding and the health of the growing infant. However, exercise and intense physical activity can raise the lactic acid concentration of breast milk, which influences the milk's taste. Therefore, women may want to breast-feed their infants before exercising.)

- **Nutrient Supplements**—During lactation, most women are able to obtain all nutrients from a healthy and balanced diet, without adding any nutrient supplement. However, some may need extra iron, as the maternal iron stores have dwindled during pregnancy and delivery. Once menstruation resumes, a lactating woman's iron requirement becomes about half that of a non-pregnant women of her age. Unless otherwise directed by a doctor, iron supplementation is not necessary.

- **Vitamins and Minerals**—Women are able to produce milk with adequate carbohydrate, protein, fat, and most minerals, even if their own supplies of these nutrients are limited. Any nutritional inadequacies reduce the quantity, but not the quality, of the breast milk. However, the milk's quality is maintained at the expense of maternal stores. Again, most women who consume a healthy and balanced diet need not worry about obtaining extra vitamins and minerals through supplementation, unless otherwise directed by their doctor.

- **Water**—It is important to keep from getting dehydrated when lactating. A good rule of thumb to go by is to consume water, milk, or fruit juices at mealtimes and when the infant nurses.

- **Limit Certain Foods**—Certain foods with strong or spicy flavors may alter the flavor of breast milk. Women who are nursing can usually eat a wide variety of nutritious foods, but if certain foods seem to be upsetting or causing the infant discomfort, these may need to be limited or eliminated altogether until the infant's reaction subsides. Appropriate substitutions can be made to ensure nutrient adequacies are met.

In summary, lactating women need to refrain from drinking alcohol, smoking, using other drugs, and from the over-use of vitamin and mineral supplements. Make sure to consume an adequate healthy and balanced diet, along with sufficient water intake, for proper milk production, which assures appropriate infant development. Simply put, when pregnant take care of yourself and the wonderful new life growing inside you!

CHAPTER 8
Infancy, Childhood, and Adolescence

Initially, infants drink only breast milk or formula; later, they begin to eat some solid foods. Using common sense in the selection of infant foods and providing a nurturing, relaxed environment will go a long way toward promoting an infant's overall health and well-being.

The first year of life is a time of phenomenal growth and development. Thereafter, a child continues to grow and change, but more slowly. However, the cumulative effects over the next decade are remarkable. When the child enters the teen years, the pace toward adulthood accelerates dramatically.

Nutrition During Infancy

Growth directly reflects nutrient intake and is an important parameter in assessing the nutrition status of infants and children. The following are the main points of energy and nutrient needs during infancy:

- **Energy Intake and Activity**—On average, a healthy infant's birth weight doubles by about five months of age and triples by one year, normally reaching 20-25 pounds. By the end of the infant's first year, growth slows considerably. An infant typically gains less than 10 pounds during the second year. Not only do infants grow rapidly, but their basal metabolic rate is amazingly high—about twice that of an adult, based on body weight. After six months, metabolic needs decline as the growth rate slows, but some of the energy that is stored by slower growth is spent in increased activity.

- **Protein**—No single nutrient is more important than protein. All of the body's cells and most of its fluids contain protein. It is the basic building material of the body's tissues. An excess of dietary protein can cause problems, especially in an infant.

Too much protein can stress the kidneys and liver, which must metabolize and excrete the excess nitrogen. The signs of protein overload include acidosis, dehydration, diarrhea, elevated blood ammonia, elevated blood urea, and fever, in some cases. These problems are not common, but have been observed in infants fed inappropriate foods, such as nonfat milk or concentrated formula.

- **Vitamins and Minerals**—Vitamin and mineral recommendations are based on the average amount of nutrients consumed by healthy infants breast-fed by well-nourished mothers. The infant's needs for most of these nutrients, in proportion to body weight, are more than double those of an adult. It is best to consult a doctor if the infant may not be getting the nutrients they need from food. Also, do not supplement an infant's diet without first talking to a doctor.

- **Water**—Water is one of the most essential nutrients for infants, as it is for everyone else. The younger the infant, the greater the percentage of the body weight which is water. During early infancy, breast milk or infant formula usually provides enough water to replace fluid losses in healthy infants. The water in an infant's body is easily lost because much of it is located outside the cells—between the cells and the vascular space. A few conditions that cause fluid loss, such as hot weather, diarrhea, or vomiting, may require supplemental water to prevent life-threatening dehydration.

Introducing Solid Foods

The high nutrient needs of infancy are met first by breast milk or formula, and then by a limited diet where foods are gradually added. Infants progressively develop the ability to chew, swallow, and digest a variety of foods. It is important to the infant's optimal growth and health that the selections of foods are appropriate for the various stages of development.

By 6 months, when most infants have the tongue-thrust reflex, it is time to introduce semi-solid foods into the diet. As the infant becomes accustomed to foods other than milk, continue with breast milk about twice a day, in addition to puréed vegetables and fruits.

The main purpose of introducing solid foods to infants is to provide nutrients that are no longer supplied adequately by the breast milk or formula. The foods chosen need to be foods that the infant is developmentally capable of handling, both physically and metabolically. This depends on the infant's readiness, which varies from infant to infant because of differences in growth rates, activity, and environment conditions.

Choice of Infant Foods

Infant foods need to be selected to provide variety and balanced nutrition. Commercial baby foods offer a wide assortment of palatable, nutritious foods in a safe and convenient form. However, homemade infant foods are just as nutritious as commercially prepared ones. The ingredients for homemade foods should be fresh, whole foods with no salt, sugar, or seasoning added. Puréed foods can be frozen in ice cube trays, providing convenient-sized blocks that can be easily thawed, warmed, and consumed by the infant. The following are points to keep in mind when choosing and preparing healthy foods for infants:

- **Foods to Provide Fat**—Since recommendations to restrict fat do not apply to children under the age of two, labels on foods for children under two do not provide information about fat. Fat information is omitted from the infant food labels in order to prevent parents from restricting fat in the infant's diet. In fact, because of their rapid growth, infants and young children need more fat than older children and adults.

- **Foods to Provide Iron**—Rapid growth demands iron. At four to six months, the infant begins to need more iron than stores, breast milk, or iron-fortified formula can provide. Infants can first receive iron from iron-fortified cereals, and later from meat or meat alternates such as legumes.

- **Foods to Provide Vitamin C**—Vegetables and fruits are the best source of vitamin C. At six months of age or older, the infant can have fruit juices. These need to be diluted with water before being given to an infant, to drink from a cup and not a bottle. Juices provide valuable nutrients, but should be used in moderation so as not to displace other foods.

- **Foods to Omit**—Sweets in any form, including baby food desserts, have no place in an infant's diet. They have no nutrients to support growth, and the extra food energy can promote obesity. Some products contain sugar alcohols such as sorbitol and should also be limited, as they may cause diarrhea. Canned vegetables can be inappropriate for infants, as they often contain too much sodium. Honey and corn syrup should never be fed to infants because of the risk of botulism—an often fatal food-borne illness caused by the ingestion of foods containing a toxin produced by bacteria that grow without oxygen. Infants and even young children cannot safely chew and swallow popcorn, whole grapes, whole beans, nuts, and hard candies. They can easily choke on these foods, a risk not worth taking.

Mealtimes with Toddlers

Eating habits developed during infancy and early childhood influence the overall attitude toward food throughout life. Providing not only balanced and healthy nutrition, but a safe, loving, and secure environment in which the child may grow and develop, plays an important role in the child's development. The following are six points or guidelines that may be helpful:

- Discourage unacceptable behavior, such as standing on the table or throwing food, by removing the toddler from the table until later, to eat in a proper manner. Be consistent and firm, not punitive. The toddler will then learn to behave when eating.
- Let toddlers explore and enjoy food, even if it means eating with fingers for a time. The skill of using utensils will come later.
- Do not force foods on toddlers. Rejecting new foods is normal, and acceptance is more likely as they become more familiar with new foods through repeated opportunities to taste them.

- Provide nutritious foods, and let toddlers choose which ones and how much they will eat. Gradually they will accept and acquire a taste for a variety of foods.
- Limit sweets. Infants, toddlers, and young children have little room for empty-calorie foods in their daily energy intake. Do not use sweets as a reward for eating meals or for good behavior.
- Do not turn the dining table into a battleground. Make mealtimes enjoyable and teach them healthy food choices and eating habits in a pleasant environment.

Sample Meal Plan for Toddlers

Breakfast:
½ cup iron-fortified breakfast cereal
¼ cup whole milk
½ cup orange juice

Midmorning Snack:
½ cup fruit juice
1-2 oz. cheese cubes
4-6 whole grain crackers

Lunch:
½ sandwich (1 slice whole wheat bread, 1 Tbsp. peanut butter, 1 Tbsp. jelly)
½ cup steamed carrots
1 cup whole milk

Midday Snack:
½ cup whole milk fruit yogurt
2 graham crackers

Dinner:
2-3 oz. chopped meat
¼ cup mashed potatoes
¼ cup steamed broccoli
¼ cup fresh strawberries

1 cup whole milk

Evening Snack:
1 cup whole milk

In summary, the primary food source for infants during the first 12 months of life is either breast milk or iron-fortified formula. At about 4 to 6 months, infants should gradually begin eating solid foods. By one year, they are drinking from a cup and are consistently eating solid foods.

Nutrition During Childhood
Energy and Nutrient Needs

Each year from age one to adolescence, a child grows taller by 2-3 inches and heavier by 5-6 pounds, on average. Growth charts provide valuable clues to a child's health, by helping track weight gain in proportion to height and determining if a child is overweight or underweight, as compared to the suggested standard.

Children's appetites begin to decrease around one year of age, consistent with the slowing of growth. However, children spontaneously vary in their food intakes, which coincide with their growth patterns, and need more food during periods of rapid growth than during slow growth. At times children may seem insatiable, and at other times may seem to live on just air and water.

It is not uncommon for a child's energy intake to vary from meal to meal. For example, if a child consumes less at one meal, they usually consume more at the next meal, and vice versa. Even so, their total daily intake remains constant. (**Side Note:** Overweight children are an exception, as they do not always adjust their energy intake accordingly and may consume food in response to external cues, disregarding hunger and satiety signals.)

Nutrients for the Growing Years

When children are still growing and are physically activity, their nutritional needs are great. Genetic background, gender, body size and shape are other factors which play a role in nutrient intake. The nutrients needed by children are the same as those needed by adults, but the amounts vary.

Carbohydrates provide energy for growing and physical activity. As children experience periods of rapid growth, their appetites expand and they may seem to be constantly eating. When growth slows, their appetites diminish and children eat less food at mealtimes. They also require fewer snacks.

Protein builds, maintains and repairs body tissue. It is especially important for growth. In the United States, most children do not suffer from a lack of dietary protein. It is important, however, to encourage children to eat two to three servings of meat, fish, poultry, or other protein-rich foods each day. Milk and other dairy products also are good protein sources for children.

Fats, like carbohydrates, provide energy for growing and for physical activity. It is important to make healthy fats a part of a growing child's diet. Unless otherwise recommended by a doctor, a child should consume healthy fats in their balanced and healthy diet.

Vitamins and minerals also support growth and development during the childhood years. The following vitamins and minerals are important to have in a child's diet, and are best if consumed from foods and not provided by supplementation.

- **Vitamin A**—When vegetable and fruit consumptions are low, children run the risk of having low intakes vitamin A.

- **Vitamins B (Thiamin, Niacin, Riboflavin and Other B Vitamins)**—These come from a variety of foods, including grain products, meat and meat substitutes, and dairy products. Generally, children do not have trouble getting adequate intakes of the B vitamins.

- **Vitamin C**—When vegetable and fruit consumptions are low, children run the risk of having low intakes of vitamin C.

- **Calcium**—Calcium, from milk and dairy products and from some dark-green, leafy vegetables, is usually sufficient in the diets of young children. As children approach the adolescent years, dietary calcium intakes don't always keep up with recommendations. Calcium is particularly important in building strong bones and teeth.

- **Iron**—Iron is an oxygen-carrying component of blood. Children need iron because of rapidly expanding blood volume during growth. For girls, the beginning of menstruation in late childhood adds an extra demand for iron, due to the regular loss of iron in menstrual blood. Meats, fish, poultry, and enriched breads and cereals are the best sources of dietary iron. Iron-deficiency anemia can be a problem for some children.

When appetites slow down and children don't seem to eat very well, concerned parents often jump at the option of using a vitamin-mineral supplement. Commonly, children don't need such supplements, but if one is being used, select a multiple vitamin and mineral supplement.

Parents should provide a variety of foods and establish regular mealtimes and snack times. In most cases, nutrient needs will be adequately met. If parents feel there is a reason to be concerned about a child's poor nutrient intake, they should consult a doctor or nutritionist.

Sample Food Serving

Whole Grain and Enriched Breads, Cereals, and Other Grain Products

Key Nutrients: Carbohydrates, Thiamin, Niacin, and Iron

Suggested Daily Servings: At least 6 servings (Include several servings of whole-grain products daily)

Serving Sizes:

- 1 slice of bread
- 1/2 hamburger bun or English muffin
- 1 small roll, biscuit, or muffin
- 3—4 small or 2 large crackers
- 1/2 cup cooked cereal, rice, or pasta
- 1 ounce of ready-to-eat breakfast cereal

Fruits Including Citrus, Melon, Berries, and Other Fruits

Key Nutrients: Carbohydrates, Vitamin A, and Vitamin C

Suggested Daily Servings: At least 2 servings

Serving Sizes:

- A whole fruit such as a medium apple, banana, or orange
- A grapefruit half
- A melon wedge
- 3/4 cup of juice
- 1/2 cup of berries
- 1/2 cup cooked or canned fruit
- 1/4 cup dried fruit

Vegetables Dark Green—Bright Red, Dry Beans, and Other Starchy Vegetables

Key Nutrients: Carbohydrates, Vitamin A, and Vitamin C

Suggested Daily Servings: At least 3 servings (Include all types regularly; use dark green, leafy vegetables and dry beans and peas several times a week)

Serving Sizes:

- 1/2 cup of cooked vegetables
- 1/2 cup of chopped raw vegetables
- 1 cup of leafy raw vegetables, such as lettuce or spinach

Meat, Poultry, Fish, and Alternates (Eggs, Dry Beans and Peas, Nuts, and Seeds)

Key Nutrients: Protein, Thiamin, Niacin, and Iron

Suggested Daily Servings: 2—3 servings

Serving Sizes:

Amounts should total 5-7 ounces of cooked lean meat, poultry, or fish a day. Count 1 egg, 1/2 cup cooked beans, or 2 tablespoons peanut butter as 1 ounce of meat.

Milk, Cheese, and Yogurt

Key Nutrients: Protein, Calcium, and Riboflavin

Suggested Daily Servings: 2 servings

Serving Sizes:

- 1 cup of milk
- 8 ounces of yogurt
- 1 1/2 ounces of natural cheese
- 2 ounces of process cheese

Fats and Sweets

Key Nutrients: Fat

Suggested Daily Servings: Choose fats and sweets to meet energy needs only after you've eaten recommended servings from the other food groups.

Serving Sizes:

- 1/2 frozen yogurt or ice cream
- 1 oatmeal raisin cookie or chocolate cookie
- 1 frozen fruit bar

Sample Meal Plan for Children

Breakfast:
½ cup cereal

½ cup 2% milk
½ banana
¾ cup orange juice

Midmorning Snack:
¼ cup trail mix (a combination of sunflower seeds, peanuts, pumpkin seeds, raisins)

Lunch:
Peanut butter and jelly sandwich (2 slices whole wheat bread, 2 Tbsp. peanut butter, 1 Tbsp. jelly)
½ cup carrot sticks
¾ cup 2% milk

Midday Snack:
6 whole grain crackers
2 oz. cheese cubes

Dinner:
2 oz. baked chicken
½ cup macaroni and cheese
¼ cup steamed broccoli
½ cup fresh grapes

Evening Snack:
1 peanut butter cookie
½ cup 2% milk

Nutrition-Related Concerns During Childhood

Most children in America and Canada are well nourished and meet their average energy intakes, which are sufficient enough to support normal growth. However, malnutrition, food allergies, obesity, and other disorders affect some children. Most can be treated with proper and adequate nutrition consumption or elimination of the allergen. The following are points that address nutrition-related concerns that occur during childhood:

- **Hunger and Malnutrition**—When hunger is chronic, children become malnourished and this causes an array of health problems within the body. The source of hunger in America is poverty. Malnourished children are not as alert and energetic as children that are healthy and are getting proper nutrition.

- **Hunger and Behavior**—Even if hunger is temporary, as when a child misses one meal, behavior and academic performance are affected. Children who eat nutritious meals and snacks throughout the day show signs of improved behavior and performance, compared to children who are unable to have meals and snacks consistently. The average child and adult should eat every 3-4 hours in order to maintain a blood glucose concentration high enough to support the activity of the brain and the rest of the nervous system. A child's brain is as big as an adult's, and the brain is the body's chief glucose consumer, using about three times as much glucose per day as the rest of the body. It is important to notice, too, that a child's liver is much smaller than an adult's. The liver is responsible for storing glucose as glycogen and releasing it into the blood as needed. A child's liver can store only about four hour's worth of glycogen, so they need to eat fairly often.

- **Food Allergies**—True food allergies occur when protein fractions of a food or other large molecules are absorbed into the bloodstream and elicit an immunologic response. (**Side Note:** Remember that proteins and other large molecules of food are normally dismantled in the digestive tract, in order to be able to be absorbed without such reaction.) The body's immune system reacts to these rather large food molecules as it does to other antigens—by producing antibodies, histamines, or other defensive agents. Allergies may have one or two components, but they always involve antibodies, which may or may not exhibit symptoms. This means that allergies can be diagnosed only by testing for antibodies. Still, symptoms exactly like those of an allergy may not be caused by one. Identifying a true food allergy requires a through health history, a physical examination, and diagnostic tests to eliminate other diseases. Once a food allergy has been diagnosed, therapy requires strict elimination of the offending food(s). Food allergies are most common during the first few years of life, but then children usually outgrow or become tolerant to the allergenic food.

- **Food Intolerances**—Not all adverse reactions to foods are food allergies. Signs of adverse reactions to foods include stomachaches, headaches, rapid pulse rate, nausea, wheezing, hives, bronchial irritation, coughs, and other such discomforts. Among the causes may be reactions to chemicals on or in foods, such as the flavor enhancer monosodium glutamate (MSG); digestive diseases, such as obstructions or injuries; enzyme deficiencies, such as lactose intolerance; and even psychological aversions. These reactions involve symptoms but no antibody production, so they are food intolerances rather than allergies.

- **Hyperactive Disorders**—Most children are naturally active and many of them become overly so on occasion. However, hyperactive children tend to have trouble sleeping or staying focused on even the simplest task, and act impulsively. Taking a look at the child's diet and making changes can be of great benefit in most cases. Eliminating sweets, processed foods, and foods that contain a lot of dye is recommended. Including more fresh whole foods like vegetables, fruits, and whole grains will aid in providing the child with adequate nutrients from sources that are tasty and appealing.

- **Obesity**—The incidence of childhood obesity has increased dramatically over the past three decades. Like their parents, children in America are becoming overweight. It is likely that children have grown more overweight because of the kinds and the quantity of foods they are consuming and the lack of physical activity. Obesity often causes psychological problems, because people judge others on appearance more than on character. Many obese children may suffer discrimination by adults and rejection by their peers. They may have a poor self-image, a sense of failure, and a passive approach to life. The initial goal for obese children is to address and treat the cause. Treatment must consider the many aspects of the problem(s) and possible solutions. An integrated approach is most effective, involving diet, physical activity, psychological support, and behavioral changes.

In summary, children's appetites and nutrient needs reflect their stage of growth. It is recommended to provide a balanced and healthy diet that has a wide variety of fresh vegetables, fruits, whole grains, and quality protein. Those who are chronically hungry and who may suffer from malnourishment usually experience growth retardation. However, when hunger is temporary and nutrient deficiencies are mild, the problems are more subtle. Childhood obesity and other health problems can be eliminated by taking the proper precautions and insuring that the child consumes a healthy and balanced diet, along with getting physical activity daily.

Nutrition During Adolescence

As children become adolescents, they continue to change in many ways. Their physical changes make their nutrient needs higher, and their emotional, intellectual, and social changes make meeting these needs a challenge at times.

Adolescences make more choices for themselves than they did as children: they are not fed, they eat; they are not sent out to play, they choose if they are going to engage in any physical activity. At the same time, there are the social pressures to either allow their bodies to develop or to focus on meeting extreme ideas of slimness or athletic prowess. If they are concerned about how diet can improve their lives, they may go on a crash diet in order to wear the latest clothing styles, stay away from greasy foods in an effort to clear up acne, or eat a large meal of spaghetti to prepare for an important sporting event.

Growth and Development During Adolescence

With the onset of adolescence, the body's continued steady growth speeds up suddenly and noticeably, and the growth patterns of females and males become distinct. Hormones are known to direct the intensity and duration of the adolescent growth spurt, profoundly affecting every organ of the body, including the brain. After about two to three years of growth, and a few more at a much slower pace, the adolescent becomes a physically mature adult. The distinct physical changes of males and females are as follows:

Males

Growth: Rapid gains around age 14, then growth slows to a stop at maturity.

Hair: Hair on forehead begins to move upward (recede); hair grows on face, under arms, and around the genitals; other body hair may grow coarser and longer.

Skin: Acne may develop.

Body Shape and Composition: Muscle tissue develops.

Hormonal Changes: Testicles produce more testosterone.

Reproductive Organs: Penis and testicles enlarge; sperm production begins; ejaculations begin.

Females

Growth: Rapid gains around age 12, then growth slows to a stop at maturity.

Hair: Hair grows under arms and genital area; other body hair may grow coarser and longer.

Skin: Acne may develop.

Body Shape and Composition: Hips widen, fat deposits collect, and breasts develop.

Hormonal Changes: Ovaries produce more estrogen and progesterone.

Reproductive Organs: Uterus and ovaries enlarge; genitals enlarge; ovum ripening begins; normal vaginal secretions begin, including a mucus-like daily secretion and monthly menstruation.

Energy and Nutrient Needs During Adolescence

Energy and nutrient needs are greater during adolescence than any other time of life, except for pregnancy and lactation. Nutrient needs rise throughout childhood, peak in adolescence, and then level off or even diminish as adolescents become adults. The following are the main points of energy and nutrient needs during adolescence:

- **Energy Intake and Activity**—The energy needs of adolescents vary greatly, depending on their gender, current rate of growth, body composition, and physical activity. Boys' energy needs tend to be especially high; they usually grow faster than girls and develop a greater proportion of lean body mass. For example, an active boy of 15 may need 4,000 calories or more a day just to maintain his weight. Girls start growing earlier than boys and attain shorter heights and lower weights, so their energy needs peak sooner and decline earlier. For example, an active girl of 15 whose growth is nearly at a standstill may need about 2,000 calories a day to maintain her weight. The insidious problem of obesity becomes ever more apparent in adolescents and often continues into adulthood. Without intervention, overweight adolescents will face numerous physical and socioeconomic consequences for years to come. The consequences of obesity are so dramatic, and society's attitude toward the obese is so negative, that teens feel compelled to lose weight, even when their weight is normal or below normal. It is always best to maintain a healthy weight by consuming a balanced and healthy diet, with moderate physical activity.

- **Vitamins and Minerals**—For most, the need for vitamins and minerals increases during the adolescent years. Several of the vitamins and minerals recommended for adolescents are similar to those for adults. However, it must be understood that the diet is to provide all the nutrients the body needs during adolescence. It is important to talk to a doctor before taking any vitamin or mineral supplements.

The RDA Energy Recommendations for Adolescents

Age: 11—14 yrs.
Calories/Day for Females: 2,200 Calories
Calories/Day for Males: 2,500 Calories

Age: 15—18 yrs.
Calories/Day for Females: 2,200 Calories
Calories/Day for Males: 3,000 Calories

Sample Meal Plan for Adolescents

Breakfast:
1 cup cereal
1 cup 1% milk
Raisin bran muffin
1 cup orange juice

Midmorning Snack:
6 whole grain crackers
2 oz. cheese cubes

Lunch:
Roast beef and cheese sandwich (2 slices whole wheat bread, 1 Tbsp. low-fat mayo, lettuce, tomato, 2 oz. roast beef, 1 oz. cheese)
½ cup carrot sticks
1 cup 1% milk

Midday Snack:
Whole grain cinnamon raisin bagel
2 oz. low-fat cream cheese

Dinner:
Spaghetti with meatballs (1 ½ cups cooked pasta and 1 cup
meat sauce)
1 cup tossed salad with 2 Tbsp. dressing
1 whole grain roll
1 cup 1% milk

Evening Snack:
¼ cup trail mix (a combination of peanuts, almonds, sunflower
seeds, pumpkin seeds, and raisins)

Healthful Food Choices
Knowing what to eat can be confusing for anyone. Everywhere
you look, there is news about what is or isn't good for you. Some basic
principles have weathered the fad diets and stood the test of time. Here
are a few tips on making healthful food choices during adolescence and
the years thereafter.

- Eat lots of vegetables and fruits. Choose from the rainbow of
  colors available to maximize variety. Eat non-starchy vegetables
  such as spinach, carrots, broccoli or green beans with meals.
- Choose whole grain foods over processed grain products. Try
  brown rice with your stir-fry or whole wheat spaghetti with
  your favorite pasta sauce.
- Include dried beans (like kidney or pinto beans) and lentils in
  your meals.
- Include fish in your meals 2-3 times a week.
- Choose lean meats, like cuts of beef that end in "loin" such as
  sirloin. Remove the skin from chicken and turkey.
- Choose low-fat dairy products such as 1% milk, low-fat yogurt
  and low-fat cheese.
- Choose water over calorie-free "diet" drinks, fruit juice instead
  of fruit punch, unsweetened tea rather than sweet tea and other
  sugar-sweetened drinks.
- Choose liquid oils for cooking instead of solid fats that can be
  high in saturated and trans fats. Remember that fats are high
  in calories. If you're trying to lose weight, watch your portion
  sizes of added fats.

- Cut back on high-calorie snack foods and desserts like chips, cookies, cakes, and full-fat ice cream.
- Eating too much of even healthful foods can lead to weight gain; watch portion sizes.

Adolescents like the freedom to come and go as they choose, and likewise, it is important to inform them of healthful food choices so that they are able to choose healthful foods as part of their daily choices. Below is a comparison of unhealthful (**Instead of This**) and healthful (**Try This**) food choices. Stick to the "**Try This**" and you will always be consuming a healthful diet, whether or not you are an adolescent.

Grains

Instead of This:

- Croissants, biscuits, and white breads and rolls
- Doughnuts, pastries, scones
- Fried tortillas
- Sugar cereals and regular granola
- Snack crackers
- Potato or corn chips, buttered popcorn
- White pasta
- White rice
- Fried rice, or pasta and rice mixes that contain high-fat sauces

Try This:

- Low-fat whole grain breads and rolls (wheat, rye, pumpernickel)
- English muffins; whole grain bagels
- Soft tortillas (corn or whole wheat); pita bread
- Oatmeal; low-fat granola; whole grain cereal
- Crackers (animal, graham, rye, soda, saltine, oyster)
- Pretzels (unsalted); popcorn (unbuttered)
- Whole wheat pasta
- Brown rice
- Rice or pasta (without egg yolk) with low-fat sauces

Vegetables and Fruits

Instead of This:

- Fried vegetables or vegetables served with cream, cheese or butter sauces
- Coconut
- French fries, hash browns, or potato chips

Try This:

- All vegetables raw, steamed, broiled, baked or tossed with a very small amount of olive oil
- Fruit (fresh or canned in light syrup)
- Baked, mashed or boiled potatoes

Meat, Poultry, and Fish

Instead of This:

- Regular or breaded fish sticks or cakes, fish canned in oil, seafood prepared with butter or served in high-fat sauce
- Prime or marbled cuts
- Pork spare ribs; bacon
- Regular ground beef
- Lunch meats such as pepperoni, salami, bologna, or liverwurst

Try This:

- Fish that is fresh, frozen, or canned in water
- Select grade lean beef (round, sirloin, loin)
- Lean pork (tenderloin, loin chop)
- Lean or extra-lean ground beef, ground chicken or turkey breast
- Lean lunch meats such as turkey, chicken and ham

Dairy

Instead of This:

- Whole or 2% milk
- Evaporated milk
- Regular buttermilk
- Yogurt made with whole milk
- Regular cheese (examples: American, Brie, cheddar, and Swiss)
- Regular cottage cheese
- Regular cream cheese
- Regular ice cream

Try This:

- Skim or 1% milk
- Evaporated skim milk
- Buttermilk made from skim (or 1%) milk
- Low-fat yogurt
- Low-fat cheese with 3-5 grams of fat per serving, including natural cheese, and nondairy cheese such as soy cheese
- Low-fat, nonfat, and dry-curd cottage cheese with less than 2% fat
- Low-fat cream cheese (no more than 3 grams of fat per ounce)
- Sorbet, sherbet, or low-fat ice cream (no more than 3 grams of fat per 1/2 cup serving)

Fats, Oils, and Sweets

Instead of This:

- Cookies
- Shortening, butter or margarine
- Regular mayonnaise
- Regular salad dressing
- Using fat (including butter) to grease pan

Try This:

- Fig bars, gingersnaps, or molasses cookies
- Olive, soybean, or canola oils
- Low-fat or light mayonnaise
- Low-fat or light salad dressing
- Nonstick cooking spray

Problems Adolescents Encounter

As adolescents continue to physically mature and grow independent, it may present a new world of choices which they will encounter on a daily basis. The consequences of those choices will influence their nutritional health both now and later in life. Some adolescents are introduced to and begin using drugs, alcohol, and tobacco; others wisely refrain from this. It is best to provide information about the use of these particular substances, because most are first exposed to them during adolescence. The following are brief summaries of substances to avoid:

- **Alcohol Abuse**—Adolescents face the decision of whether to drink alcohol, and even though the law forbids the sale of alcohol to those under 21 years of age. Though, most adolescents who seek alcohol can and will obtain it. Alcohol provides energy but no nutrients, and it can displace nutritious foods from the diet as well. No matter what age one is, alcohol is a deadly substance and has no nutrient value for the body.

- **Drug Abuse**—The nutrition problems associated with various drugs, whether they are over-the-counter drugs or more harmful substances like cocaine, vary in degree. Those who abuse drugs in general face multiple nutrition problems, and during withdrawal from drugs, it is important to identify, treat, and correct these nutrition problems. Far too often, adolescents get involved with various drugs that are deemed harmful to the body even in small doses. It is vital that we keep such substances away from adolescents and adults alike, as they harm the body.

- **Smoking**—It has been reported that nearly half of American adolescents smoke cigarettes at one time or another. The effects of cigarette smoking go beyond the scope of nutrition, but smoking influences hunger, body weight, and nutrient status. Smoking a cigarette eases the feelings of hunger. When a smoker receives a hunger signal, they tend to choose a cigarette instead of food to quiet their hunger. This kind of behavior ignores the body's natural signals and postpones energy and nutrient intake, leading to a weight loss. This is why smokers tend to weigh less and to gain weight more easily when they give up smoking. Smokers are more likely to have lower intakes of dietary fiber, vitamin A, beta-carotene, folate, and vitamin C. Having low intakes of vegetables and fruits rich in these nutrients is noteworthy, considering their protective effect against lung cancer and so on.

In summary, nutrient needs rise rather dramatically as children head into the next phase of rapid growth and change—the adolescent years. In addition to learning to make wise food choices, adolescents need to refrain from using substances that will impair their overall health, both now and in the future.

Eating Disorders During Adolescence

Eating is controlled by many factors, including appetite, food availability, family, peers, cultural practices, and attempts at voluntary control. Dieting to a body weight leaner than needed for health is highly promoted by current fashion trends, sales campaigns for special foods, and in many activities and professions. Eating disorders involve serious disturbances in eating behavior, such as extreme and unhealthy reduction of food intake or severe overeating, as well as "purging" unwanted calories through self-induced vomiting, exercising, or laxative and diuretic abuse. Feelings of distress or extreme concern about body shape, size or weight are common.

Eating disorders are not due to a failure of will or behavior. They are real, treatable disorders in which certain maladaptive patterns of eating take on a life of their own. The main types of eating disorders are anorexia nervosa, bulimia nervosa, and binge-eating (compulsive overeating) disorder. Eating disorders frequently develop during adolescence and tend to continue into adulthood, if not treated.

What Is an Eating Disorder?

An eating disorder is a serious medical problem in which a sufferer becomes totally preoccupied with weight and exhibits severe eating behaviors. These behaviors can range from eating massive quantities of food to starving oneself. Often developing in adolescence or early adulthood, eating disorders can also occur during childhood or later in adulthood. These disorders include:

- **Anorexia nervosa**—Basically, this is self-starvation. Persons with anorexia have a distorted body image, viewing themselves as overweight even when they are dangerously thin. They may exhibit intense fear of gaining weight, and often deny the seriousness of their current weight loss or low body weight. Often they eat barely enough food to survive—for example, a single slice of dry toast all day. Some will also exercise excessively as a way of burning dreaded calories.
- **Bulimia nervosa**—This involves episodes of binge eating followed by attempts to purge the body of food due to fear of anticipated weight gain. People who have this disorder may have a normal weight. Even their closest relatives may not be aware of their behavior, which may involve vomiting food after meals or taking dangerous quantities of laxatives.
- **Binge-eating disorder**—This involves frequent episodes of overeating without purging. A binge eater may wake up at night to secretly raid the refrigerator, or binge publicly.

While these are the primary eating disorders, there are others. These include: purging without binging, anorexic behavior with a less severe weight loss, and chewing and spitting out food without actually swallowing or purging.

Young women are the primary sufferers of eating disorders, but men are diagnosed, too. In fact, an estimated 5-15 percent of those with either anorexia or bulimia and an estimated 35 percent of those with binge-eating disorders are male. Binge-eating disorder seems to affect men and women equally.

More Than Just Food

Eating disorders rarely involve just food. People often use food as a coping mechanism to help them feel in control when feelings or situations seem overwhelming. Starving, for example, is a way for those with anorexia to feel more in control of their lives, which ultimately eases their tension, anger, and anxieties. The same is true for those with bulimia.

People with a negative body image have a greater likelihood of developing an eating disorder and are more apt to suffer from feelings of depression, isolation, low self-esteem, and obsessions with weight loss.

Why Do Eating Disorders Occur?

The reasons are complex, and no single factor is to blame. Clearly, our thin-obsessed culture in the United States plays a part. Despite the professional and societal advances women have made in the last few decades, many still define themselves primarily by their appearance and how physically attractive they are. The pressure is on to be thin.

But for most people with eating disorders, the reasons are more complex than simply societal pressures. People who feel helpless, worthless, or have poor self-esteem are more likely to suffer, as are those who are depressed or have anxiety disorders.

Stressful life events can also contribute to the onset of an eating disorder. These can include moving to a new city, starting a new job, divorce, or the death of a loved one.

Researchers are studying the possibility of a genetic connection to eating disorders. They are also examining the effect of brain chemicals on the development of eating disorders.

Detecting an Eating Disorder

Detecting an eating disorder can be difficult. The symptoms—limiting food intake, compulsively exercising, and expressing unhappiness with body weight—are frequently considered normal in our culture. Many who engage in these behaviors may not feel they have a problem at all. However, it is easy for these habits to spin out of control and become a potentially life-threatening eating disorder.

If left untreated, or if a given treatment is not effective, eating disorders can cause serious physical problems, including low blood sugar, pancreas and liver damage, heart failure, osteoporosis, heart rhythm problems, thought impairment, and ultimately death.

Signs of Eating Disorders

The signs of eating disorders in adolescents and adults are:

- A preoccupation with weight, counting calories, grams and dieting
- Body weight less than 85 percent of the proper normal range
- A refusal to eat certain foods, such as carbohydrates
- Frequent remarks about feeling fat or overweight despite weight loss
- A denial of hunger
- Intense fear of gaining weight or of becoming fat, even though underweight
- Regular excuses to avoid mealtimes or social situations involving food
- Development of rituals involving food, e.g., eating foods in a certain order or excessive chewing
- Excessive exercise regimen, despite the weather, fatigue, illness, or injury
- Withdrawal from normal friends and activities

Unfortunately, adults and adolescents suffering from eating disorders may find it uncomfortable to even admit to themselves that they have a problem, much less seek help from a trained professional. It is important to be aware of a life-draining disorder and to help those who are suffering from one before it is too late.

In summary, many adolescents engage in self-destructive eating behaviors in order to meet unsuitable weight standards for their body. Anorexia, bulimia, and compulsive overeating deceive adolescents with empty promises of fixing their problems and soothing insecurities. All the while, they are stripping away their identity and sense of worth in a desire to fit in and be accepted. Eating disorders are a harrowing addiction, which affect adolescents physically, mentally, emotionally and spiritually.

Early detection of an eating disorder may prevent years of significant misery and disruption in an adolescent's life. How is your child's diet?

CHAPTER 9
Adulthood and the Later Years

Good nutrition is vital for everyone as they move through different stages of life. The amount and type of food needed varies with age, gender, levels of activity, as well as during pregnancy and breast-feeding. A healthy diet and lifestyle in adulthood helps to prevent or slow the progression of chronic diseases, such as heart disease, osteoporosis, stroke, diabetes, and some cancers. A healthy diet and lifestyle also helps to ensure you will be fit, full of energy, have healthy teeth, skin and hair, and a good body weight.

Throughout the course of life, the mind and body is constantly undergoing changes. On a biological level, the major organs—heart, lungs, eyes, ears, and brain—lose a portion of their functioning ability as one grows older. On a psychological level, changes in short-term memory may decrease the ability to recall information that was just spoken. Aging also affects the social environment. Upon retirement, friends may elect to move to a warmer climate or nearer to family or friends. Friendship patterns may change from those centered around a work life to those centered around religion, travel, clubs or organizations, or volunteer activities.

All in all, not only does aging affect the body and mind, it also affects the nutritional status.

Nutrition During Adulthood and Beyond

For adults (ages 18 to 50 and beyond), weight management is a key factor in achieving health and wellness. In order to remain healthy, adults must be aware of changes in their energy needs, based on their level of physical activity, and balance their energy intake accordingly.

An adult individual needs to balance energy intake with his or her level of physical activity to avoid storing excess body fat. Dietary practices and food choices are related to wellness and affect health, fitness, weight management, and the prevention of chronic diseases such as osteoporosis, cardiovascular diseases, cancer, and diabetes.

At the onset of adulthood, it is very important to keep the energy intake in check, and to make sure that all of the nutritional needs are met. This can be accomplished by ensuring that an adequate amount of energy is consumed. This will vary in each individual, because of the degree of activity, physical fitness, and weight. Foods that are chosen to provide the energy must be highly nutritious, containing high amounts of essential nutrients such as vitamins, minerals, and essential proteins.

Energy and Nutrient Needs During Adulthood

On average, it is estimated that adult energy needs decline about 5 percent per decade. One reason is that adults usually reduce their physical activity as they age, although they need not do so. Another reason is that lean body mass—muscle—diminishes, slowing the basal metabolic rate.

The lower energy expenditure of adults requires that their intake be less in order to maintain a healthy weight. Normally, energy intakes decline in parallel with the body's needs. Not all adults are overweight, but many are, which indicates that their food intake has not declined to compensate for their change in lifestyle. Being overweight adults increases the risk for numerous diseases and can cause complications for those who suffer from disabilities or life-threatening health problems.

Whether an adult is overweight or maintaining a healthy weight, it is important that they consume a balanced and healthy diet which provides enough nutrients to adequately meet their body's needs. The following is a summary of the nutrients that are important for all stages of life, and it clarifies what is most essential to include in a balanced and healthy diet.

- **Carbohydrates and Fibers**—Abundant carbohydrates are needed to protect protein from being used as an energy source. Complex carbohydrates such as whole grains, vegetables, fruits, and legumes provide an excellent source of fiber and essential vitamins and minerals. A diet that emphasizes fiber-rich foods, along with protein and fat, tends to provide all the nutrients the body needs.

- **Proteins**—Now that energy needs have decreased, protein must be obtained from low-calorie sources of high-quality protein. Such as lean meats, poultry, fish, and eggs, as well as low-fat dairy products and legumes. Protein is important as adults age, because it aids in the support of a healthy immune system and helps to prevent muscle wasting.

- **Fats**—As is true during all stages of life, fat needs are to be limited, but not eliminated. Consuming healthy fats in moderation may help prevent or delay the development of cancer, heart disease, or other degenerative diseases.

Important Vitamins and Minerals for Adults

Most adults are able to obtain adequate vitamin and mineral intakes simply by including foods from all food group sources in a balanced and healthy diet. However, some adults tend to abstain from certain food groups for one reason or another, thinking that they do not need them. For example, some may omit vegetables and fruits altogether while consuming all the sweets and desserts they want.

Some adults may need to add vitamins and/or minerals through supplements or fortified foods in order to meet their nutritional needs. Again, food is the best source of vitamins and minerals. However, vitamin and mineral supplements are sometimes needed to contribute to overall nutrient intakes. In most cases, taking a daily multivitamin and mineral supplement may be all that is needed. The following are nutrients that adults sometimes lack in their diets:

- **Vitamin B 12**—Healthy adults should be able to obtain the vitamin B-12 from a balanced diet. Red meat, poultry, fish, eggs, and milk products provide the majority of vitamin B-12 in the diet.

- **Vitamin D**—Vitamin D is necessary for the intestines to absorb dietary calcium. Vitamin D comes from food and is also produced by the skin when exposed to sunlight. Fish, fortified dairy products, and cereal products provide the majority of vitamin D in the diet.

- **Calcium**—Calcium is a building block for bone. Adequate dietary calcium intake is one of the most important factors for maintaining healthy bones and bone strength, but is not always sufficient to fully protect against the rapid bone loss that can occur. Vegetables and dairy products provide the majority of calcium in the diet.

- **Magnesium**—Not only is magnesium needed in order to properly absorb and use calcium in the body, but it has many other important uses in the body as well. Low magnesium (hypomagnesemia) is often associated with low calcium (hypocalcemia) and potassium (hypokalemia) levels. Deficiency of magnesium causes increased irritability of the nervous system with tetany (spasms of the hands and feet, muscular twitching and cramps, spasm of the larynx, etc.). Vegetables, whole grains, legumes, and nuts provide the majority of magnesium in the diet.

- **Iron**—Iron is necessary for the transport of oxygen (via hemoglobin in red blood cells) and for oxidation by cells (via cytochrome). Deficiency of iron is a common cause of anemia. It is best to obtain iron needs from food sources such as meat, poultry, eggs, vegetables, and cereals. Red meats, poultry, and fish, as well as plant foods such as lentils and beans, provide the majority of iron in the diet.

- **Zinc**—Zinc is an essential mineral that is found in almost every cell. It stimulates the activity of approximately 100 enzymes, which are substances that promote biochemical reactions in the body. Zinc supports a healthy immune system, is needed for wound healing, helps maintain the senses of taste and smell, and is needed for DNA synthesis. Zinc also supports normal growth and development during pregnancy, childhood, and adolescence. Red meat and poultry provide the majority of zinc in the diet. Other good food sources include seafood, whole grains, beans, dairy products, and nuts.

Sample Meal Plan for Adults

Breakfast:
1 cup whole grain cereal
1 cup 1% milk
1 banana

Midmorning Snack:
1 whole grain bagel with 1 oz. low-fat cream cheese

Lunch:
Roast beef and cheese sandwich (2 slices whole grain bread, 1 Tbsp. low-fat mayo, 1 tsp. mustard, lettuce, tomato, 2 oz. roast beef, 1 oz. cheddar cheese)
1 apple
Tea

Midday Snack:
6-8 whole grain crackers
1 cheese stick

Dinner:
Stir-Fry (2 oz. sautéed meat and 1 cup sautéed mixed vegetables)
¾ cup wild rice
Tossed salad with low-fat dressing

Evening Snack:
1 cup frozen yogurt with ½ cup granola

The Aging Process

Some things you never outgrow—like the need for healthful eating. Good nutrition is important at every stage of life, from infancy through late adulthood. The basics of a balanced diet remain the same, but individual nutritional needs change as you grow older. No matter what your age, it is never too late to start living a healthier life.

Whether you are 50 or 85, active or homebound, your food choices will affect your overall health in the years ahead. The risk for certain diseases associated with aging—such as heart disease, osteoporosis and diabetes—can be reduced with a lifestyle that includes healthy eating. Good nutrition also helps in the treatment and recovery from illness. While healthy living can't turn back the clock, it can help you feel good longer.

Eating a balanced and healthy diet means consuming a variety of foods each day. During different stages of life, for one reason or another, the body may not be getting the right amounts of nutrients. There are several factors that indicate an increased risk for poor nutrition during the later years of adulthood. If three or more of the risk factors listed below are true in your life, consult a doctor or a nutritionist:

- Ill health
- Poor eating habits
- Unexpected weight gain or loss
- Taking medications that interfere with food
- Poor dental health
- Economic hardship
- Loneliness and lack of social contacts
- Inability to care for yourself

Older adults need the same nutrients as younger people, but in differing amounts. As you get older, the number of calories needed is usually less than when you were younger. This is because basic body processes require less energy when there is a decline in physical activity and loss of muscle. Contrary to popular belief, basic nutrient needs do not decrease with age. In fact, some nutrients are needed in increased amounts. The challenge is to develop a balanced eating plan that supplies plenty of nutrients but not too many calories.

This can be done by choosing nutritious foods that are low in fat and high in fiber, like whole grain breads and cereals, vegetables, and fruits. Also, be sure to include moderate amounts of low-fat dairy products and protein foods like meat, poultry, fish, beans, and eggs. Sweets and other foods high in sugar, fat, and calories can be enjoyed from time to time, but the key is to eat them sparingly.

Special Considerations for Older Adults

Nutrition through the prime years of adulthood may play a greater role than has been realized in preventing many changes, which once were thought to be inevitable consequences of growing older. The following points highlight some of the obstacles that older adults may encounter as they age, and recommendations on how to correct or help minimize the changes that are bound to occur.

- **Smell and Taste**—The ability to smell and taste may decline gradually with age. When the sense of smell becomes dulled, it affects the sense of taste and makes food less appetizing. Also, some medications may leave a bitter taste, which affects saliva, giving foods a bad flavor. Smoking reduces the ability to enjoy flavors, too. Poor eating habits can result when food just doesn't taste as good as it used to. To compensate for the loss of smell and taste, create meals that appeal to all the senses. Intensify the taste, smell, sight, and texture of foods. Perk up flavors with herbs, spices and lemon juice rather than relying solely on salt or sugar. Choose foods that look good and have a variety of textures and temperatures. Try new ideas. Use garlic and other seasoning on foods, add a new texture (like crushing crackers in soup), or change the temperature (such as serving applesauce warm with cinnamon).

- **Dry Mouth**—Dry mouth is another problem faced by many older adults. When your mouth feels like it is filled with cotton balls and your lips are parched and cracked, food just doesn't taste good. It can be difficult to chew and swallow because of a lack of saliva. Dry mouth is a potential side effect of many medications, such as drugs to lower blood pressure or treat depression. It may also be a symptom of cancer or kidney failure. To relieve dry mouth discomfort, watch out for spicy foods that irritate the lips and tongue. Eat soft foods that have been moistened with sauces or gravies. Try sucking on hard candies or popsicles and drink plenty of fluids. A room humidifier may help by moistening the air. It will also help if you breathe through your nose, not your mouth.

- **Tooth Loss**—Tooth loss or mouth pain can be an obstacle to good eating. Generally, people who wear poorly fitting dentures chew 75 percent to 85 percent less efficiently than those with natural teeth. Dentures should be adjusted for a proper fit. Softer foods are easier to chew. Drinking plenty of water or other fluids with meals may make swallowing easier. Good dental care (brushing, flossing, regular check-ups) will help keep teeth and gums healthy.

- **Loss of Appetite**—Many older adults say they just aren't hungry. There are many factors that influence appetite, including digestive problems, certain medications, depression or loneliness. To encourage eating and appetite, keep portions small, allow plenty of time to dine, eat smaller meals more often, prepare attractive meals, play music, eat meals with friends, and increase physical activity where possible. Consult a physician if the lack of appetite results in unwanted weight loss.

- **Constipation**—Constipation can be a chronic problem for many older adults. It can be caused by not getting enough fiber or fluids and by being physically inactive. To stay regular and avoid the strain of constipation, engage in physical activity, drink plenty of fluids, and eat fiber-rich foods such as whole grain breads and cereals, legumes, vegetables and fruit. Fiber gives bulk to stools and fluids help keep stools softer, making them easier to eliminate.

- **Trouble Digesting Milk**—Some older adults have trouble digesting milk, even if it wasn't a problem in their younger years. The small intestine may no longer be producing the enzyme lactase, which breaks down the natural sugar (lactose) in milk. If the lactase enzyme is missing, you may experience bloating, abdominal cramps and diarrhea. Tolerance to lactose is variable. Try eating smaller amounts of these foods, eating them during a meal instead of alone, or having them less often (perhaps every other day). Lactose-reduced and lactose-free products are now available. Also, the lactase enzyme is available in tablets or drops that can be added to milk before drinking it.

- **Medications**—It seems that many older adults are on one or more medications. In some circumstances, medications can improve health and quality of life, but some can profoundly affect nutritional needs. Be sure to consult with a doctor or pharmacist as to specific instructions concerning food-drug interactions and directions on when and how to take medications.

- **Socializing with Others**—Part of the pleasure of eating is in socializing with others. Many older adults who live alone may find mealtimes boring or depressing. Put some fun back into eating by getting together with friends for weekly or monthly potluck dinners. Look for a senior center in your community. This is a great way to meet old friends and make new ones, and many centers have programs that offer a midday meal on weekdays. Take advantage of early-bird specials or senior discounts at restaurants, and don't hesitate to take home a doggie bag. Invite a friend to lunch at your home. Join a community service club or organization. Many of these groups plan social activities that often include getting together for meals. When home alone, make meals a special event with candles, a tablecloth, music, and something delicious to eat. Look to local agencies that help older adults who find it hard to cook their own meals or get out of the house. Meals-On-Wheels programs provide food for people who are homebound. Home health care organizations can provide aides who will shop and prepare meals for older disabled adults. Some local churches or community groups have volunteers who will help older adults with shopping and food preparation.

Aging is an inevitable and natural process, which is programmed into the genes at conception. However, by consuming a balanced and healthy diet, and engaging in physical activity, the process can be more enjoyable.

In summary, it may seem obvious, but eating right is one of the first steps in living a healthy life. Consuming a balanced and healthy diet provides the nutrients and energy for the body to survive, so it makes sense to eat the right foods. But most individuals in today's hurried world don't take time to eat regular nutritious meals. The body can only take so much abuse, and by the time mid to late adulthood comes around, most are experiencing health problems that need not be part of their lives. Eat to take care of your body as we all want to live a healthy and comfortable life!

PART 3
Weight Management

CHAPTER 10
Overweight

Despite the preoccupation with body image and weight loss, the prevalence of overweight and obesity in America continues to rise dramatically. If you are very overweight, you are more likely to develop heart disease or a stroke than if you are lean. You are also more likely to have high blood pressure and high cholesterol, both risk factors for heart disease in their own right. High levels of blood fats and high blood pressure favor the formation of fatty plaques in arteries, which, combined with "sticky blood" and an increased tendency to form clots, present a high risk of blood clots. Blood clots in the coronary arteries can affect the supply of blood to the heart, which can lead to a heart attack. Being overweight also makes you more prone to developing diabetes, gallstones, arthritis, and certain types of cancer. The good news is that by choosing to make changes in your lifestyle and losing some weight, you could reduce the risk of developing these conditions. Even a modest and permanent weight loss of 5-10 percent will cut your risk of heart disease; the added bonus is a new, healthier and fitter you! However, before going further, it is helpful to understand the development and metabolism of body fat in the body.

Fat Cell Development

When more energy is consumed than is spent, much of the excess energy is stored in the fat cells of adipose tissue. The amount of fat in an individual's body reflects both the number and the size of fat cells. The number of fat cells increases rapidly during the growing stages of late childhood and early puberty. Fat cell numbers increase more rapidly in obese children than lean children, and obese children entering their teen years might already have as many fat cells as do adults of normal weight.

Fat cells expand in size as they fill with fat droplets. As fat cells reach their maximum size, they tend to also divide. Therefore, obesity begins to develop when an individual's fat cells increase in number, in size, or both. It is possible to shrink fat cells that already exist, but you are not able to cause the fat cells to break down and disappear. Individuals with extra fat cells have a tendency to regain lost weight rapidly; with weight grain, their fat cells readily become filled. Thus, prevention of becoming overweight is most critical during the growing years, when the fat cells are increasing in number.

Fat Cell Metabolism

It is known that the enzyme lipoprotein lipase (LPL) promotes fat storage in both adipose and muscle cells. Individuals with high LPL activity store fat more easily, because LPL is mounted on fat cell membranes. Overweight individuals have much more LPL activity in their fat cells than lean individuals.

The activity of LPL is regulated by gender-specific hormones—estrogen in women and testosterone in men. In women, fat cells in the breasts, hips, and thighs produce abundant LPL, putting fat away in those body sites. In men, fat cells in the abdomen produce abundant LPL. This enzyme activity explains why men tend to develop central obesity, whereas women more readily develop lower-body fat.

The enzyme activity may explain why some individuals who lose weight so easily regain it. After weight loss, LPL activity increases, and it does so most efficiently in individuals who have been heavy prior to weight loss. Apparently, weight loss serves as a signal to the gene that produces the LPL enzyme. Individuals easily regain weight after having lost it because they are battling against enzymes that want to hold on to and store fat. This also explains the observation that there is an inner mechanism that seems to regulate an individual's weight or body composition at a fixed point; the body works to adjust and restore the set point. (**Side Note:** Differences are also apparent in the activity of the enzymes controlling fat breakdown in various parts of the body. The lower body is less active than the upper body in releasing fat from storage.)

Set-Point Theory

There are many internal physiological variables—such as blood glucose, blood pH, and body temperature—in order for the body to remain fairly stable under a variety of conditions. Though the hypothalamus and other regulatory centers continually monitor and delicately adjust conditions so as to maintain homeostasis, the stability of such complex systems may depend on set-point.

Research has confirmed that after weight gains or losses, the body works to adjust its metabolism so to restore the original weight. Energy expenditure increases after weight gain and decreases after weight loss. These changes in energy expenditure differ from those expected and based on body composition, and help to explain why it is difficult for an underweight individual to maintain weight gain and for an overweight individual to maintain weight loss.

In summary, fat cells tend to develop by increasing in number and size. Preventing excessive weight gain depends on maintaining a reasonable number of fat cells. With gains or losses, the body will attempt to return to its previous set-point.

Defining Overweight and Obesity

Overweight and obesity are both labels for ranges of weight that are greater than what is generally considered healthy for a given height. The terms also identify ranges of weight that have been shown to increase the likelihood of certain diseases and other health problems.

For adults, overweight and obesity ranges are determined by using weight and height to calculate a number called the Body Mass Index (BMI). (**Side Note:** See how to calculate your BMI in chapter 12.) BMI is used because, for most individuals, it correlates with their amount of body fat.

- An adult who has a BMI between 25 and 29.9 is considered overweight.
- An adult who has a BMI of 30 or higher is considered obese.

It is important to remember that although BMI correlates with the amount of body fat, it does not directly measure body fat. As a result, some individuals (such as athletes) may have a BMI that identifies them as overweight, even though they do not have excess body fat. Other methods of estimating body fat and its distribution include measurements of skin fold thickness and waist circumference, calculation of waist-to-hip circumference ratios, and techniques such as ultrasound, computer tomography, and magnetic resonance imaging (MRI).

For children and teens, BMI ranges above a normal weight have different labels (at risk of overweight and overweight). Additionally, BMI ranges for children and teens are defined so that they take into account normal differences in body fat between boys and girls and differences in body fat at various ages.

Causes of Obesity

Overweight and obesity are a result of energy imbalance over a long period of time. The cause of energy imbalance for each individual may be due to a combination of several factors. Individual behaviors, environmental factors, and genetics all contribute to the complexity of the obesity epidemic. Genetics and the environment may increase the risk of an individuals weight gain. However, the choices an individual makes in eating and physical activity also contributes to overweight and obesity. Behavior can increase an individual's risk for gaining weight. The following are explanations of some of the contributing factors leading to obesity:

- **Calorie Consumption**—In America, a changing environment has broadened food options and eating habits. Grocery stores stock their shelves with a greater selection of products. Pre-packaged foods, fast-food restaurants, and soft drinks are also more accessible. While such foods are fast and convenient, they also tend to be high in fat, sugar, and calories. Choosing many foods from these areas may contribute to an excessive calorie intake. Some foods are marketed as healthy, low-fat, or fat-free, but may contain more calories than the fat-containing food they are designed to replace. It is important to read food labels for nutritional information and to eat in moderation. Portion size has also increased. Many individuals may be eating more during a meal or as a snack because of larger portion sizes. This results in increased calorie consumption. If the body does not burn off the extra calories consumed from larger portions, fast-food, or soft drinks, weight gain can occur.

- **Calories Used**—The body needs calories for daily functions such as breathing, digestion, and daily activities. Weight gain occurs when calories consumed exceed this need. Physical activity plays a key role in energy balance because it uses up calories consumed. Regular physical activity is good for overall health. Physical activity decreases the risk for colon cancer, diabetes, and high blood pressure. It also helps to control weight; contributes to healthy bones, muscles, and joints; reduces falls among the elderly; and helps to relieve the pain of arthritis. Physical activity does not have to be strenuous to be beneficial. Moderate physical activity, such as 30 minutes of brisk walking five or more times a week, also has health benefits. Despite all the benefits of being physically active, most Americans are sedentary. Technology has created many time- and labor-saving products. Some examples include cars, elevators, computers, and dishwashers. Individuals use cars to run short-distance errands instead of walking or riding a bicycle. As a result, these recent lifestyle changes have reduced the overall amount of energy expended in everyday life. The belief that physical activity is limited to exercise or sports may keep people from being active. Another myth is that physical activity must be vigorous to achieve health benefits. Physical activity is any bodily movement that results in an expenditure of energy. Moderate-intensity activities such as household chores, gardening, and walking can also provide health benefits.

- **Environment**—Individuals may make decisions based on their environment or community. For example, an individual may choose not to walk to the store or to work because of a lack of sidewalks. Communities, homes, and workplaces can all influence individuals health decisions. Because of this influence, it is important to create environments that make it easier to engage in physical activity, and to eat a healthy diet.

- **Genetics**—Science shows that genetics plays a role in obesity. Genes can directly cause obesity in disorders such as Bardet-Biedl syndrome and Prader-Willi syndrome. However, genes do not always predict future health. Genes and behavior may both be needed for an individual to be overweight. In some cases, multiple genes may increase the susceptibility for obesity and require outside factors, such as an abundant food supply or little physical activity.

- **Diseases and Drugs**—Some illnesses may lead to obesity or weight gain. These include Cushing's disease and polycystic ovary syndrome. Drugs such as steroids and some antidepressants may also cause weight gain. A doctor is the best source to determine whether illnesses, medications, or psychological factors are contributing to weight gain or are making weight loss difficult.

In summary, obesity has many causes and combinations of causes in different individuals. Some causes, such as overeating and physical inactivity, may be within the individual's control.

Reasonable Treatments of Obesity

Obesity is associated with increased disease and mortality. Weight loss reduces risk factors for complications associated with the excess weight, including diabetes and cardiovascular diseases. There are several treatment options for the management of overweight and obese individuals, including diet therapy, changes in physical activity, behavioral therapy, drug therapy, surgery, and a combination of these.

The initial goal of weight loss therapy is to decrease body weight by about 10 percent. Once this goal is met, then further weight loss can be attempted. This weight loss will not occur overnight, but you can see a difference within mere weeks if you stay with your program. Once the weight is lost, maintenance needs to be implemented to ensure that the weight stays off.

Diet Therapy

Lifestyle modifications, such as increasing physical activity and decreasing calorie intake, are recommended instead of dieting. Crash diets should definitely be avoided. The best approach to changing your diet is to talk to your doctor and find out what is best for you. Your doctor can provide you with dietary guidelines or refer you to a dietician for further help. Dietary guidelines will differ for each person depending on height, weight, concurrent health conditions, and desired amount of weight loss. A diet must be established that will both allow for weight loss and be easy to comply with. Maintenance of your program is the key to keeping the pounds off.

Exercising is important to any good weight loss program. An aerobic exercise program reduces weight, regardless of any changes you make in your diet. Adding 45 minutes of aerobic exercise a day is the equivalent of losing 400-800 calories, depending on the intensity. Minimally, that would result in losing one pound per week. Even if you can only exercise three times per week, that would still help you lose almost 2 pounds per month, or 20 pounds over a year! Remember that this is without any changes in your diet. Eliminating 500 calories a day from your diet (the equivalent of one large order of French fries) will double your results.

Weight training and calisthenics also help you to reduce weight— not by direct loss, but by decreasing fatty tissue and increasing lean body mass. This will increase metabolism, and the body will burn more calories while at rest.

Obese patients should start slowly with low-intensity walking or swimming, and advance intensity as tolerated. If you have cardiovascular disease or other conditions that may make exercise very difficult, talk to your physician before you begin.

Behavioral Therapy

Behavior modification is common to all weight loss programs. Modification includes strategies that aid individuals to overcome barriers to comply with dietary changes and physical activity. Most behavioral modification programs encourage self-monitoring of both diet and exercise to increase one's own awareness of the activities. Modification strategies may also include stress management, social support, and stimulus control.

Combining behavioral therapy, diet therapy, and increased physical activity should be considered as the initial method for weight loss. This combination should be continued for at least 6 months before proceeding to drug therapy.

Drug Therapy

After all other modes of losing weight have failed, you should talk to your physician about your options with drug therapy. For some individuals, drug therapy may be considered as a supplement to a comprehensive weight loss program that also includes diet, exercise, and behavioral therapy. Medications can be used to stimulate weight loss by either decreasing the appetite or by inhibiting the absorption of fat from the intestines.

Many health food and supplement stores promote various "natural" or herbal products for weight loss. Even though they claim to be effective and natural, these products can be associated with certain harmful side effects. The U.S. Food and Drug Administration (FDA) has stringent rules pertaining to the safety, efficacy, and quality that pharmaceutical manufacturers must follow in order to market drugs in the U.S. Manufacturers of herbal supplements do not have to follow these same rules to sell their products. For this reason, there is limited research evaluating supplements' safety and efficacy in the human body. As a result, anyone who chooses to take these substances does so at their own risk.

In summary, the most important thing to remember is that weight loss takes time and effort, and is a lifelong process. Also, it is important to set reasonable goals. Sensible weight loss does not occur overnight, and it takes major changes in your lifestyle before significant changes in weight may be observed. Permanent weight loss can be reached by continued lifestyle changes.

Sample Meal Plan for Weight Loss

Breakfast:
1 cup whole grain cereal
1 cup 1% milk
1 banana

Midmorning Snack:
5 whole grain crackers
1 oz. cheese stick

Lunch:
Turkey and cheese sandwich (2 slices whole grain bread, 1 Tbsp. low-fat mayo, 1 tsp. mustard, lettuce, tomato, 2 oz. turkey, 1 oz. cheddar cheese)
1 cup carrot sticks

Tea

Midday Snack:
Apple slices with 2 Tbsp. peanut butter

Dinner:
1 ½ cups vegetable soup
2 cups tossed salad with low-fat dressing
1 whole grain roll

Evening Snack:
1 granola bar
1 cup 1% milk

In summary, the key to losing weight is being consistent in eating smaller portions, choosing healthful foods, and making time for three meals, plus two or three snacks. The question still remains though, are you over weight and if so what are you doing about it?

CHAPTER 11
Underweight

Being underweight, like being overweight, is based on a healthy weight for a given height and sex. An individual can be regarded as moderately underweight if he or she weighs 10 percent below a healthy body weight, and markedly so if the weight is 20 percent below a healthy weight range.

Individuals are considered underweight if their Body Mass Index (BMI) falls below a certain threshold. (**Side Note:** See how to calculate your BMI in chapter 12.) Again, BMI is a measure determined by an individual's age, height, and weight. For infants and children, a BMI below the 10th percentile for a specific age indicates an individual who is underweight. For adults, a BMI below 18.5 for females and 20.5 for males is considered underweight. A BMI of 17.5 indicates an individual is very underweight.

It is widely known that Individuals who are underweight are at high risk for malnutrition. Being underweight can affect growth and development, and it can cause infertility or delayed menstruation. It can also result in fatigue, irritability, and a lack of concentration, and can impair the body's ability to thermoregulate itself. Due to a decreased immune response, underweight individuals are less resistant to infections and disease.

Problems of Underweight

Being underweight is defined as having a BMI of less than 18.5, and can occur with anorexia nervosa or other eating disorders, from loss of appetite, or from illness. Many chronic medical conditions, cancers, and infections can also result in weight loss to the point of being underweight. Being underweight is linked to menstrual irregularity (which can lead to infertility) and osteoporosis in women, and to a greater risk of early death in both women and men.

Many individuals—especially women—are concerned about body weight, even when their weight is actually normal. Excessive concern about weight may cause or lead to unhealthy behaviors, such as excessive exercise, self-induced vomiting, and the abuse of laxatives or other medications. These practices may only worsen the concern about weight.

Unexplained weight loss is sometimes an early clue to a health problem. If you lose weight suddenly when you're not attempting to reduce, or you lose weight for unknown reasons, visit your doctor to determine if a medical condition is responsible for the weight loss.

Causes of Underweight

While most individuals are concerned about losing excess pounds, some have the opposite problem—how to add pounds onto an extra-thin body. Genetics may be an important factor in the inability to gain weight. Other causes may be inadequate nutrition or excessive athletic activity. In some cases, persistent weight loss can be a sign of a mood or eating disorder, a digestive disorder such as malabsorption, endocrine problems such as thyroid disease, or cancer.

If you are unable to maintain or gain weight, it is important to see a doctor so that you may have a complete medical work-up, to see if there are any underlining causes going on within the body. The most common causes of being underweight are as follows:

- Insufficient calorie intake
- Unhealthy eating habits like skipping meals, and frequent fasting
- Metabolic disorders
- Presence of intestinal worms
- Chronic diarrhea
- Diabetes
- Inadequate digestion
- Heredity

Weight Gain Strategies

To gain weight, it may be necessary to change eating habits in order to meet the caloric demands on the body. Instead of eating to satisfy taste buds or hunger, it is recommend that you eat foods at times when you are not hungry, and throughout the day. It costs 3,500 calories to gain one pound. In order to gain one pound a week, you have to consume 500 extra calories every day. Here are some tips for getting those extra calories daily in a balanced and healthy meal plan.

- **Eat Frequently**—Make time for 3 large meals and 2-3 hefty snacks every day.

- **Eat Larger Portions**—Consume larger than normal portions at meals.

- **Eat Higher Calorie Foods**—Choose dried fruit, starchy vegetables, dense whole grains, hearty bean soups, and plain nuts.

- **Eat Healthy Fats**—Add healthy unsaturated fats: olive and canola oil, nuts, seeds, peanut butter, avocados.

- **Add Healthy Extras**—Honey, jam, dried fruit, wheat germ, nonfat dried milk powder, whey or soy protein powder. (**Side Note**: Nutritional supplements should be considered. There are commercially prepared high-protein and high-calorie food supplements available.)

- **Exercising to Build Muscle**—To gain weight, use strength training primarily and increase energy intake to support exercise. Another 500-700 calories are needed in order to support both exercise and the building of muscle.

In summary, the incidence of being underweight and the health problems associated with it are less prevalent than being overweight and the problems associated with that. In order to gain weight, an individual must increase their energy intake by selecting energy-dense foods, and eating regular meals. It is also beneficial to take in larger portions and consume extra snacks. As well as, incorporate exercise such as strength training.

Sample Meal Plan for Weight Gain

Breakfast:
1 ¼ cups granola
¼ cup raisins
1 ½ cups 2% milk
1 cup orange juice

Midmorning Snack:
1 cinnamon raisin bagel with 2 oz. low-fat cream cheese

Lunch
Tuna pita sandwich (7-inch pita pocket, 1 6.5 oz. can tuna, 4
Tbsp. low-fat mayo, lettuce, tomato, sprouts)
1 apple, cut into slices
1 ½ cups lentil soup

Midday Snack:
½ cup trail mix (a combination of sunflower seeds, peanuts,
pumpkin seeds, and raisins)
1 cup 2% milk

Dinner
2 cups spaghetti
1 ½ cups tomato basil pasta sauce
¼ cup parmesan cheese
2 cups tossed salad with olive oil vinaigrette dressing
1 whole grain rolls with 1 Tbsp. butter

Evening Snack:
Peanut butter and jelly sandwich (2 slices whole wheat bread, 2
Tbsp. peanut butter, 1 Tbsp. jelly)
1 cup 2% milk

In summary, the key to gaining weight is being consistent in eating
larger than normal portions, choosing healthful high-calorie foods, and

making time for three meals, plus two or more hefty snacks. Do you know someone who is trying to gain weight?

CHAPTER 12
Energy Balance and Body Composition

The body has been designed to cope with many extremes, but for the most part, there is a constant energy balance which the body operates on. An adequate, balanced, and healthy diet must satisfy the body's needs for energy and all essential nutrients. Furthermore, dietary energy needs and recommendations cannot be considered in isolation from other nutrients in the diet, as the lack of one will influence the others.

Energy Balance

The body's energy requirements are estimated from measures of energy expenditure plus the additional energy needs for growth, pregnancy and lactation. Recommendations for dietary energy intake from food must satisfy these requirements for the attainment and maintenance of optimal health, physiological function, and well-being. The latter (well-being) depends not only on health, but also on the ability to satisfy the demands imposed by society and the environment, as well as all the other energy-demanding activities that fulfill individual needs.

Energy balance is achieved when input (i.e., dietary energy intake) is equal to output (i.e., total energy expenditure), plus the energy cost of growth in childhood and pregnancy, or the energy cost to produce milk during lactation. When energy balance is maintained over a prolonged period, an individual is considered to be in a steady state. This can include short periods during which the day-to-day balance between intake and expenditure does not occur. An optimal steady state is achieved when energy intake compensates for total energy expenditure and allows for adequate growth in children, and pregnancy and lactation in women, without imposing metabolic, physiological, or behavioral restrictions that limit the full expression of an individual's biological, social, and economic potential.

Within certain limits, humans can adapt to transient or enduring changes in energy intake through possible physiological and behavioral responses related to energy expenditure and/or changes in growth. Energy balance is maintained, and a new steady state is then achieved. However, adjustments to low or high energy intakes may sometimes entail biological and behavioral penalties, such as reduced growth velocity, loss of lean body mass, excessive accumulation of body fat, increased risk of disease, forced rest periods, and physical or social limitations in performing certain activities and tasks. Some of these adjustments are important and may even increase the chances of survival in times of food scarcity. The following definitions are based on the assumption that requirements for energy will be fulfilled through the consumption of a diet that satisfies all nutrient needs.

- **Energy Requirement**—The amount of food energy needed to balance energy expenditure in order to maintain body size, body composition, and a level of necessary and desirable physical activity consistent with long-term good health. This includes the energy needed for the optimal growth and development of children, for the growth of tissues during pregnancy, and for the secretion of milk during lactation consistent with the good health of mother and child.

- **The Recommended Level of Dietary Energy Intake**—For a population group, this is the mean energy requirement of the healthy, well-nourished individuals who constitute that group. Based on these definitions, a main objective for the assessment of energy requirements is the prescription of dietary energy intakes that are compatible with long-term good health. The levels of energy intake recommended by this expert consultation are based on estimates of the requirements of healthy, well-nourished individuals. It is recognized that some populations have particular public health characteristics that are part of their usual, normal life. Foremost among these are population groups in many developing countries, where there are numerous infants and children who suffer from mild to moderate degrees of malnutrition and who experience frequent episodes of infectious diseases, mostly diarrhea and respiratory infections. Special considerations are made in this report for such sub-populations.

- **Daily Energy Requirements and Energy Intakes**—Energy requirements and recommended levels of intake are often referred to as daily requirements or recommended daily intakes. These terms are used as a matter of convention and convenience, indicating that the requirement represents an average of energy needs over a certain number of days, and that the recommended energy intake is the amount of energy that should be ingested as a daily average over a certain period of time. There is no implication that exactly this amount of energy must be consumed every day, or that the requirement and recommended intake are constant, day after day. Neither is there any biological basis for defining the number of days over which the requirement or intake must be averaged. As a matter of convenience, taking into account that physical activity and eating habits may vary on some days of the week, periods of seven days are often used when estimating the average daily energy expenditure and recommended daily intake.

- **Average Requirement and Inter-Individual Variation**—Estimates of energy requirements are derived from measurements of individuals. Measurements of a collection of individuals of the same gender and similar age, body size, and physical activity are grouped together to give the average energy requirement—or recommended level of dietary intake—for a class of people or a population group. These requirements are then used to predict the requirements and recommended levels of energy intake for other individuals with similar characteristics, but on whom measurements have not been made. Although individuals in a given class have been matched for characteristics that may affect requirements—such as gender, age, body size, body composition, and lifestyle—there remain unknown factors that produce variations among individuals.

Components of Energy Requirements

Energy for the metabolic and physiological functions of humans is derived from the chemical energy found in food and its macronutrient constituents (i.e., carbohydrates, proteins, and fats), which act as fuel for the body to function and operate properly. After food is ingested, its chemical energy is released and converted into thermic, mechanical, and other forms of energy. The following procedures continually take place in the body to provide energy at one time or another:

- **Basal Metabolism**—This comprises a series of functions that are essential for life, such as: cell function and replacement; the synthesis, secretion and metabolism of enzymes and hormones to transport proteins and other substances and molecules; the maintenance of body temperature; uninterrupted work of cardiac and respiratory muscles; and brain function. The amount of energy used for basal metabolism in a period of time is called the Basal Metabolic Rate (BMR). It is measured under standard conditions that include being awake and in the supine position after 10-12 hours of fasting and 8 hours of physical rest, and being in a state of mental relaxation in an ambient environmental temperature that does not elicit heat-generating or heat-dissipating processes. Depending on age and lifestyle, BMR represents 45-70 percent of daily total energy expenditure, and it is determined mainly by the individual's age, gender, body size, and body composition.

- **Metabolic Response to Food**—Eating requires energy for the ingestion and digestion of food and for the absorption, transport, interconversion, oxidation and distribution of nutrients. These metabolic processes increase heat production and oxygen consumption, and these processes are known by terms such as dietary-induced thermogenesis, specific dynamic action of food, and thermic effect of feeding. The metabolic response to food increases total energy expenditure by about 10 percent of the BMR over a 24-hour period in individuals eating a mixed diet.

- **Physical Activity**—This is the most variable and, after BMR, the second largest component of daily energy expenditure. Humans perform obligatory and discretionary physical activities. Obligatory activities can seldom be avoided within a given setting, and they are imposed on the individual by economic, cultural, or societal demands. The term "obligatory" is more comprehensive than the term "occupational," because in addition to occupational work, obligatory activities include daily activities such as going to school, tending to the home and family, and other demands made on children and adults by their economic, social, and cultural environment.

- **Discretionary Activities**—Although not socially or economically essential, these activities are important for health, well-being, and a good quality of life in general. They include the regular practice of physical activity for fitness and health; the performance of optional household tasks that may contribute to family comfort and well-being; and the engagement in individually and socially desirable activities for personal enjoyment, social interaction, and community development.

- **Growth**—The energy cost of growth has two components: 1) the energy needed to synthesize growing tissues, and 2) the energy deposited in those tissues. The energy cost of growth is about 35 percent of total energy requirements during the first 3 months of age. This cost falls rapidly to about 5 percent at 12 months and about 3 percent in the second year. It remains at 1-2 percent until mid adolescence and is negligible in the late teens.

- **Pregnancy**—During pregnancy, extra energy is needed for the growth of the fetus, placenta, and various maternal tissues— such as in the uterus, breasts, and fat stores—as well as for changes in maternal metabolism and the increase in maternal effort at rest and during physical activity.

- **Lactation**—The energy cost of lactation has two components: the energy content of the milk secreted; and the energy required to produce that milk. Well-nourished lactating women can derive part of this additional requirement from body fat stores that were accumulated during pregnancy.

Calories In and Calories Out

What happens inside the body when you eat too much or too little food? The body ends up with an unbalanced energy budget, meaning you have taken in more or less food energy than you spent. When more food energy is consumed than is needed, excess fat enters the fat cells in the body's adipose tissue for storage. When the energy supplies run low, stored fat is withdrawn. The daily energy balance can therefore be stated like this:

Change in Energy Stores = Energy in Energy Out

The energy in foods and beverages is the only contributor to the "energy in" side of the energy balance equation. Before an individual can decide how much food energy they need in a day, they must first become familiar with the amounts of energy in foods and beverages. As an example of calories associated with food portions: an apple gives you about 125 calories from carbohydrates; a regular candy bar gives you about 250 calories, mostly from fat and simple carbohydrate. Though the energy present in a serving of food or in a day's meals can easily be estimated, no easy method exists for estimating how much energy an individual spends or how much the body needs. Many authorities have published recommended energy intakes for various age-sex groups in their populations, and these can be found with a little effort. These figures are good for population studies, but energy needs vary so widely among individuals that it is impossible to estimate a person's energy needs without knowing the facts about their characteristics, such as their basal metabolism and their lifestyle. The recommendations for energy intake are based on average individuals. For example, an intake of 2,200 calories per day is recommended for a woman who is assumed to be 20 years old, standing 5'5" tall, weighing about 128 pounds, of average body fatness, and engaging in light activity. The man needing 2,900 calories per day is a healthy 20-year-old of average body fatness that stands 5'10" tall, weighs 160 pounds, and is also lightly active. Taller individuals need proportionately more energy than shorter people to balance their energy budgets because their greater surface area allows more energy to escape as heat. Older people generally need less than younger people, due to slowed metabolism and reduced muscle mass that occurs partly because of reduced physical activity. On average, the energy need diminishes by 5 percent per decade beyond age 30.

In reality, though, no individual is average, and their energy needs vary widely. In any group of 10 or 20 similar individuals with similar activity levels, one may expend twice as much energy per day as another. A 60-year-old who bikes, swims, or jogs each day may need as many calories as another person of 30. Clearly, with such a wide range of variation, a necessary step in determining any individual's energy need is to study them.

One way to estimate energy needs is to monitor food intake and body weight over a period of time in which activities are typical of the individual's lifestyle. By keeping an accurate record of all the foods and beverages consumed for a week or two, and if weight has not changed during the past few months, it can be concluded that the energy budget is balanced. At least three days of honest record-keeping are necessary because intakes fluctuate from day to day. A week or two of records are better still.

Another method of determining energy needs is based on energy output. To estimate output an individual must compute the amount of the two major components of energy expenditure, and then they are added together. This method leaves out a third energy component—the body's metabolic response to food. About 5-10 percent of a meal's energy value is used in stepped-up metabolism in the 5 or so hours after the meal. This category of energy expenditure is called the thermic effect of food. Although this amount of energy could affect expenditures over the long run, most experts believe its effects are negligible. The two major ways in which the body spends energy are to fuel its basal metabolism, and to fuel its voluntary activities. Basal metabolism generates energy to support the body's work, which goes on all the time without our conscious awareness. Reactions such as breathing, heartbeat, thinking, digesting, and cell division all require energy, and the amount of energy needed to fuel these activities is what determines the basal metabolism.

Basal metabolism consumes a surprisingly large amount of fuel, and the basal metabolic rate (BMR) varies from individual to individual. An individual whose total energy needs are 2,000 calories a day may spend as many as 1,200-1,400 of them to support basal metabolism (doing no voluntary activity). The hormone thyroxine directly controls basal metabolism. The fewer hormones secreted, the lower the energy requirements for basal functions; the more hormone produced, the higher the energy requirements. Thyroxine is produced by the thyroid gland, and proper amounts of iodine are necessary for its production. Many other factors also affect the BMR.

Nearly everyone wants to know how they can speed up their metabolism to promote fat loss. You cannot speed up your BMR in the space of just a few days. However, it is possible to amplify the second component of energy expenditure—voluntary activities. This occurs when more calories are spent. And if this continues day after day, the BMR will also increase. Lean tissue is more metabolically active than fat tissue, so a way to speed up the BMR to the maximum possible rate is to make endurance and strength-building exercise a daily habit in order for body composition to become as lean as possible.

As for fuel for voluntary activities, the amount of energy spent in exercise depends somewhat on personal style and on having the right amounts of all the proper nutrients the body needs to get through these activities. In general, the heavier the weight of the body parts that move during exercise and the longer the time that is invested, the more calories are spent. The leaner the body becomes, the more calories are spent through basal metabolic functions.

In summary, an individual takes in energy from food and, on average, spends most of it on basal metabolic activities, some of it on physical activities, and a little on the thermic effect of food. Since energy requirements vary from individual to individual, such factors as age, gender, and weight must be considered when calculating energy spent on basal metabolism. The intensity and duration of the activity must be taken into account when calculating expenditures on physical activities.

Calculating the BMR

The factors are different for men and women because men generally have more muscle tissue. For example, for a 150-pound woman, her BMR would be calculated as follows:

1. Change pounds to kilograms: 150 pounds/2.2 pounds per kilogram = 68 kilograms
2. Multiply weight in kilograms by the BMR factor: 68 kilograms X 0.9 calories per kilogram per hour = 61 calories per hour
3. Multiply the calories used in one hour by the hours in a day: 61.2 calories per hour X 24 hours per day = 1,469 calories per day

1.0 calorie per kilogram (2.2 lbs.) of body weight per hour for men

0.9 calories per kilogram (2.2 lbs.) of body weight per hour for women

(**Side Note**: Use the same formula for men, only use 1 calorie per hour, instead of 0.9 calories.)

Determine Lifestyle:

Sedentary—Sitting down most of the day, and driving or riding whenever possible. A person who does small amounts of cooking or housework, or types at a computer, would be considered sedentary.

Light Activity—Moving around some of the time, such as a teacher might during working hours, a foreman at a factory, a salesperson in a store, and housework taking more than an hour or so continuously.

Moderate Activity—Engaging in some intentional exercise, such as an hour of jogging four or five times a week, or your occupation calls for some physical work.

Heavy Activity—A job that requires much physical labor, such as a roofer, carpenter, or construction worker. More intentional exercise than that described in moderate activity, including strength training.

Exceptional Activity—The exceptional category is reserved for those few who spend many hours a day in intense physical training, such as college or professional athletes.

The second component of energy expenditure and physical activity is calculated by multiplying the BMR calories by a percentage that varies by activity level (the levels above). These percentages are estimates or approximations of energy expenditure based on the amount of muscular work an individual typically performs during the day.

Multiply your BMR by the numbers below:

Sedentary:
Men—25-40 percent
Women—25-35 percent

Light:
Men—50-70 percent
Women—40-60 percent

Moderate:
Men—65-80 percent
Women—50-70 percent

Heavy:
Men—90-120 percent
Women—80-100 percent

Exceptional:
Men—130-145 percent
Women—110-130 percent

Calculate Total Energy Requirements:

Calculate energy expenditure using both the upper and lower ends of the range of percentages given for gender and activity level. Suppose the 150-pound woman used in the earlier example bikes about ten minutes a day, and walks to complete errands, but otherwise sits or does light housework most of the day. She would fall into the light activity category, so to estimate the range of energy she needs by multiplying her BMR calories per day by both 40 percent and 60 percent:

1,469 calories per day X 0.40 = 588 calories per day

1,469 calories per day X 0.60 = 881 calories per day

The woman needs between 588-881 calories per day to fuel voluntary activities. Total the metabolic and activity components, first using the lower number for activity energy, then using the higher number. In one day, the woman in our example spends either:

1,469 + 588 = 2,057 calories

1,469 + 881 = 2,350 calories

Estimate the woman's needs as a range of rounded values: 2,000-2,400 calories per day.

Body Weight, Body Composition, and Health

Weight gains and losses tell nothing about how the body's composition may have changed, yet weight is the measure most individuals use to judge their "fatness." For most individuals, overweight means over fat, but this is not always the case. Athletes with dense bones and well-developed muscles may be overweight by some standards, but have little body fat. Conversely, inactive individuals may seem to have acceptable weights, when, in fact, they may have too much body fat.

Defining Healthy Body Weight

Calculating BMI is one of the best methods for individual assessment of a healthy body weight. Because calculation requires only height and weight, it is inexpensive and easy for health professionals and for the general public to use. The use of BMI allows individuals to compare their own weight status to that of the general population.

Current standards for a healthy body weight are based on an individual's weight in relation to height, which is referred to as the Body Mass Index (BMI). Although weight measures are inexpensive, easy to take, and accurate, they fail to reveal two valuable pieces of information in assessing disease risk—how much of the weight is fat and where the fat is located.

BMI is calculated the same way for both children and adults. The calculation is based on the following formulas:

Measurement Units Kilograms and Meters (or Centimeters)

Formula/Calculation

Formula: weight (kg) / [height (m)]2

Calculation: [weight (kg) / height (m) / height (m)]

With the metric system, the formula for BMI is weight in kilograms divided by height in meters squared. Since height is commonly measured in centimeters, divide height in centimeters by 100 to obtain height in meters.

Example: Height = 165 cm (1.65 m), Weight = 68 kg

Calculation: 68 ÷ (1.65)2 = 24.98

Pounds and Inches

Formula/Calculation

Formula: weight (lb) / [height (in)]2 x 703

Calculation: [weight (lb) / height (in) / height (in)] x 703

Calculate BMI by dividing weight in pounds (lbs) by height in inches (in) squared and multiplying by a conversion factor of 703.

Example: Weight = 150 lbs, Height = 5'5" (65")

Calculation: [150 ÷ (65)2] x 703 = 24.96

For adults 20 years old and older, BMI is interpreted using standard weight status categories that are the same for all ages and for both men and women. For children and teens, on the other hand, the interpretation of BMI is both age and sex specific. (**Side Note**: Although the BMI number is calculated the same way for children and adults, the criteria used to interpret the meaning of the BMI number for children and teens are different from those used for adults. For children and teens, the BMI has a more defined age and sex-specific percentiles for two reasons: the amount of body fat changes with age, and the amount of body fat differs between girls and boys.)

The standard weight status categories associated with BMI ranges for adults are shown as follows:

BMI Weight Status:

- Below 18.5 = Underweight
- 18.5—24.9 = Normal
- 25—29.9 = Overweight
- 30—65 = Obese

The correlation between the BMI number and body fatness is fairly strong; however, the correlation varies by sex, race, and age. These variations include the following examples:

- At the same BMI, women tend to have more body fat than men

- At the same BMI, older people, on average, tend to have more body fat than younger adults

- Highly trained athletes may have a high BMI because of increased muscularity rather than increased body fatness

It is also important to remember that BMI is only one factor related to risk for disease, when assessing an individual's likelihood of developing overweight or obesity related diseases.

The BMI ranges are based on the relationship between body weight and disease and death. Overweight and obese individuals are at increased risk for many diseases and health conditions, including:

- Hypertension
- Dyslipidemia (for example, high LDL cholesterol, low HDL cholesterol, or high levels of triglycerides)
- Type 2 diabetes
- Coronary heart disease
- Stroke
- Gallbladder disease
- Osteoarthritis
- Sleep apnea and respiratory problems
- Some cancers (endometrial, breast, and colon)

In summary, the body mass index (BMI) is a fast and, for the most part, an effective way to measure weight and keep track of it.

Body Fat and Its Distribution

The ideal amount of body fat depends partly on the individual. A normal weight man may have from 12-20 percent body fat; a woman, because of her greater quantity of essential fat, 20-30 percent. The following are points about body fat, its distribution in the body, and tips for overall health.

- **The Criterion of Health**—In asking what is the ideal weight, individuals often mistakenly turn to fashion for the answer. It is important to keep in mind that fashion is fickle—body shapes that society values change with time, and fashion has little to do with health. The criterion for determining how much a person should weigh and how much body fat a person needs is health. Ideally, an individual has enough fat to meet basic bodily functions, but not so much as to incur health risks. In general, health problems develop when body fat exceeds 22 percent in young men; 25 percent in men over the age of 40; 32 percent in young women; and 35 percent in women over the age of 40.

- **Some Individuals Need More**—A higher percentage of body fat is probably beneficial for individuals who live in cold climates, because fat provides an insulating blanket to prevent excessive loss of body heat. A woman that becomes pregnant needs sufficient body fat to support conception and fetal growth. Going below a certain threshold for body fat, hormone synthesis falters, and individuals may become infertile, develop depression, experience abnormal hunger regulation, and become unable to keep warm. These thresholds differ for each function and for each individual as well.

- **Some Individuals Need Less**—For athletes, a lower percentage of body fat may be ideal for performance—just enough fat to provide fuel, insulate and protect the body, assist in nerve impulse transmissions, and support normal hormone activity. For some athletes, the ideal body fat might be 5-10 percent for men and 15-20 percent for women.

- **Fat Distribution**—The distribution of fat on the body may be more critical than the amount of fat alone. The intra-abdominal fat that is stored around the organs of the abdomen is referred to as central obesity or upper-body fat. It is independent of total body fat, which is associated with increased risks of heart disease, stroke, diabetes, hypertension, and some forms of cancer. Abdominal fat is common in women past menopause and even more common in men. Even when total body fat is similar, men have more abdominal fat than either premenopausal or postmenopausal women. But regardless of menopausal status, the risk of cardiovascular disease and mortality are increased for women with abdominal fat, just as they are for men. In fact, individuals who are overweight, but who do not have excessive fat around the abdomen, are less susceptible to health problems than overweight individuals with central obesity.

In summary, the ideal amount of body fat varies from individual to individual, but research has found that body fat in excess of 22 percent for young men and 32 percent for young women poses health risks. Central obesity, in which excess fat is distributed around the core of the body, presents greater health risks than excess fat distributed throughout the body.

Health Risk Associated with Body Weight and Body Fat

Body weight and fat distribution correlate with disease risks, and most individuals with a BMI between 18.5 and 29.5 have few health risks. The risk increase as BMI falls below or rises above this range. This indicates that both too little and too much body fat impairs health. (**Side Note**: Factors such as blood pressure or smoking habits raise health risks independently of BMI.) Individuals who are underweight or overweight carry a higher risk of early death than those whose weights fall within an acceptable range. The following are brief summaries of health risks associated with body weight and body fat:

- **Health Risks of Underweight**—Some underweight people enjoy an active, healthy life, but others are underweight because of malnutrition, illnesses, or unhealthy habits. Weight and fat measures alone would not reveal these underlying causes, but a complete assessment that included diet and medical history, physical examination, and biochemical analysis would. An underweight individual, especially an older adult, may be unable to preserve lean tissue during the fight against a wasting disease, such as cancer or a digestive disorder, especially when the disease is accompanied by malnutrition. Without adequate nutrient and energy reserves, an underweight individual will have a particularly hard time dealing with such medical stresses. In fact, many individuals with cancer die, not from the cancer itself, but from malnutrition. On another subject, underweight women develop menstrual irregularities and become infertile. Exactly how infertility develops is unclear, but contributing factors include not only body weight, but also restricted energy and fat intake, and depleted body fat stores. Underweight women can improve their chances of having a healthy infant by gaining weight prior to conception, during pregnancy, or both. Being underweight or having a significant weight loss is also associated with osteoporosis and bone fractures in women. For all these reasons and more, underweight individuals benefit from enough of a weight gain to provide an energy reserve and protective amounts of all the nutrients that can be stored.

- **Health Risks of Overweight**—Having excessive body fat poses such high health risks that it has been declared a disease: obesity. Being obese increases your risks of many health problems, including heart disease, stroke, diabetes, hypertension, high cholesterol levels, certain types of cancer, gout, and gallbladder disease. Being overweight can also cause problems such as sleep apnea (interrupted breathing during sleep) and osteoarthritis. The more overweight you are, the more likely you are to have health problems. These health risks can be avoided by adopting a balanced and healthy diet, getting reasonable exercise, and maintaining a healthy weight. Furthermore, overweight but fit individuals have lower risks than normal-weight, unfit individuals. A healthy weight depends on both good nutrition and moderate exercise.

- **Cardiovascular Disease**—The relationship between obesity and cardiovascular disease risk is very strong, with links to both blood cholesterol and blood pressure. Central obesity may raise the risk of heart attack and stroke as much as the three leading factors—high blood cholesterol, hypertension, and smoking. In addition to body fat and its distribution, weight gain also increases the risk of cardiovascular disease. Weight loss will effectively lower both blood cholesterol and blood pressure in obese individuals. Of course, lean and normal-weight individuals may also have high blood cholesterol and blood pressure, and these factors are just as dangerous in lean individuals as in those who are obese.

- **Cancer**—The risk of some cancers increases with both body weight and weight gain, but researchers do not fully understand the relationship. One possible explanation may be that obese individuals have elevated levels of hormones that could influence cancer development. For example, adipose tissue is the major site of estrogen synthesis in women. Obese women have elevated levels of estrogen, and estrogen has been implicated in the development of cancers of the female reproductive system. These account for about half of all cancers in women, and these types include cancer of the uterus, gallbladder, cervix, ovary, breast, and colon. Men are at greater risk for developing cancer of the colon, rectum, and prostate.

- **Diabetes**—Non-insulin-dependent diabetes mellitus (type 2 diabetes) is the most common type of diabetes in America. Type 2 diabetes reduces the body's ability to control blood sugar levels. It is a major cause of early death, heart disease, kidney disease, stroke, and blindness. Obese individuals are twice as likely to develop type 2 diabetes as individuals who are not overweight. It is possible to reduce the risk of developing this type of diabetes by losing weight and by increasing physical activity. For those who have type 2 diabetes, losing weight and becoming more physically active can help control blood sugar levels. And if you are using medicine to control blood sugar levels, weight loss, and physical activity, may make it possible to decrease the amount of medication that is needed.

In summary, the weight appropriate for an individual depends largely on factors specific to that individual, including body fat distribution, family health history, and current health status. Both the underweight and overweight extremes carry clear risks to overall health.

PART 4
Recipes for Healthful Eating

CHAPTER 13
Healthy Grocery List

Now is a good time to start making a committed effort to shopping for healthful foods and to start making home-cooked meals. In order to accomplish this, you must begin with the finest and freshest ingredients. The following are tips for adding a health advantage when grocery shopping:

The Buying Basics

- **Baked Goods**—Select products that are fresh and minimally processed, such as whole grain breads, rolls, bagels, and English muffins. Limit or omit processed cakes, pies, pastries, and doughnuts.

- **Deli**—Select lean sliced turkey, chicken, roast beef, ham, and low-fat cheeses. Limit or omit high-fat, high-sodium processed meats, including sausages, salami, bacon, and hot dogs.

- **Dairy**—Select low-fat varieties of all dairy products, including milk, buttermilk, yogurt, cottage cheese, ricotta cheese, cheese, sour cream, cream cheese, ice cream, and frozen yogurt. Limit or omit full-fat dairy products.

- **Meats**—Select meats that are lean and trimmed of visible fat. These include round, loin, sirloin, extra-lean ground beef, or tenderloin; leg or shoulder pork; skinless turkey or chicken; fresh fish and shellfish.

- **Nonperishable Foods**—Select foods that are not processed and have very few or no additives, such as canned vegetables, fruits, and beans in water or their own juices.

- **Produce**—Vegetables and fruits contain no fat or cholesterol, and are full of healthy fiber. Select the freshest and most colorful produce possible for maximum nutritional benefits.

- **Frozen Products**—Select foods that are not processed and have very few or no additives. These include vegetables, fruits, bagels, bread, low-fat ice cream, fruit bars, and some pre-made meals. Limit or omit processed frozen foods that are high in fat or have many additives.

- **Beverages**—Select bottled water. Limit or omit sodas, alcoholic beverages, and most fruit juices.

When grocery shopping, take the time to look at the products you are about to purchase. Are they really going to be of benefit to the body? Is a better choice possible? If so, buy the better choice; your body will thank you for it. Let's go shopping!

Healthy Shopping List

Complex Carbohydrates

- Oatmeal (old-fashioned or quick oats)
- Sweet Potatoes (yams)
- Beans (pinto, black, kidney)
- Oat Bran Cereal
- Granola
- Brown Rice
- Farina (Cream of Wheat)
- Multigrain Hot Cereal
- Pasta
- Rice (white, jasmine, basmati, Arborio, wild)
- Potatoes (red, baking, new)
- Whole Grain Breads, Bagels, Rolls

Fibrous Carbohydrates

- Green Leafy Lettuce
- Broccoli
- Asparagus
- String Beans
- Spinach
- Bell Peppers
- Brussels Sprouts
- Cauliflower
- Celery
- Spinach

Other Produce & Fruits

- Cucumbers
- Green or Red Peppers
- Onions
- Garlic
- Tomatoes
- Zucchini
- Fruit: Bananas, Apples, Grapefruit, Peaches, Strawberries, Blueberries, Raspberries
- Lemons or Limes

Proteins

- Chicken Breast (skinless)
- Tuna (water packed)
- Fish (salmon, sea bass, halibut)
- Extra-Lean Ground Beef or Ground Round
- Protein Powder
- Protein Bars
- Egg Whites or Eggs
- Ribeye Steaks or Roast
- Top Round Steaks or Roast (stew meat, London broil, stir-fry)
- Top Sirloin

- Beef Tenderloin (filet)
- Top Loin (New York strip steak)
- Flank Steak
- Eye of Round (cube meat, stew meat, 95% Lean Ground Round)
- Turkey Breast (skinless)

Healthy Fats

- Natural-Style Peanut Butter
- Olive Oil or Safflower Oil
- Nuts (raw peanuts, almonds, cashews, etc.)
- Flaxseed Oil

Dairy & Eggs

- Low-fat cottage cheese
- Low- or Non-fat Milk
- Low-fat cheese
- Low-fat yogurts
- Eggs

Beverages

- Bottled Water
- Green Tea
- Tea
- Natural Fruit Juices
- Natural Vegetable Juices
- Sports Drinks

Condiments & Misc.

- Low-fat Mayonnaise
- Reduced Sodium Soy Sauce
- Reduced Sodium Teriyaki Sauce
- Balsamic Vinegar
- Salsa

- Chili Powder
- Mrs. Dash
- Steak Sauce
- Maple Syrup
- Honey
- Fruit Spread
- Chili Paste
- Mustard
- Extracts (vanilla, almond, etc.)
- Low Sodium Broth (beef or chicken)
- Plain or Reduced Sodium Tomato Sauce, Puree, and Paste

CHAPTER 14
Rise and Shine Breakfasts

Remember, the body has been fasting through the night and is ready for a balanced and healthy meal to break the fast; hence, the word *breakfast*.

However, the body needs more than just a piece of toast and a cup of coffee to get going in the morning. When you grab toast and coffee, you are depriving the body of the carbohydrates, proteins, and fats it needs. Instead of rushing through an unhealthy breakfast, or no breakfast at all, take time to plan simple and quick breakfasts that will meet your body's needs and prepare it for the demands you put on it.

Try the following breakfast ideas, a different one every day, for a great variety of ways to get your day started right!

Orange Vanilla French Toast

Serves 4

4 eggs, lightly beaten
2 tsp. vanilla extract
1 ½ cups low-fat milk
¼ cup orange juice
1 tsp. cinnamon
8 slices whole wheat bread
Fresh honey or maple syrup

1. Beat together eggs, vanilla extract, milk, orange juice, and cinnamon.
2. Preheat a skillet with canola oil over medium-high heat. Once it is hot, dip the bread into the liquid mixture.
3. Gently place the bread in the skillet and let it cook until golden brown on both sides.
4. Place two slices of French toast on a plate and drizzle with some fresh honey or maple syrup.

Serving Suggestion:
Serve with fresh citrus slices and milk.

Strawberry Breakfast Smoothie

Serves 4

2 cups frozen strawberries
2 scoops vanilla protein powder
2 cups low-fat milk
2 eggs
1 Tbsp. honey
2 Tbsp. flaxseed oil

1. Place all ingredients in a blender and blend until smooth.
2. Pour into four tall glasses and enjoy.

Serving Suggestion:
Serve with a toasted whole grain bagel.

Scrambled Egg Burritos

Serves 4

8 10-inch flour tortillas
8 eggs, lightly beaten
1 tsp. salt
¼ tsp. pepper
1 ½ cups low-fat cheddar cheese, shredded
1 cup salsa

1. Heat a skillet over medium-high heat. Place each tortilla in the skillet and soften for 15 seconds; turn over for another 15 seconds. Wrap heated tortillas in foil to keep warm.
2. Beat eggs with salt and pepper.
3. Add oil to warm skillet; pour in eggs and cook until scrambled.
4. Place a portion of eggs, salsa, and cheese on each tortilla and wrap burrito-style. Serve on a plate.

Serving Suggestion:
Serve with fresh melon slices.

Hot Oat Pancakes

Serves 4

4 egg whites
1 cup low-fat ricotta cheese
2 Tbsp. canola oil
1 tsp. vanilla extract
2/3 cup old-fashioned oats, uncooked
¼ tsp. salt
1 tsp. baking powder
Fresh honey or fruit syrup

1. Heat a large skillet coated with canola oil over medium-high heat.
2. Measure the egg whites, ricotta, oil, vanilla, oats, salt, and baking powder into a blender or food processor; blend for 5-6 seconds.
3. Spoon 2 Tbsp. of the batter into the skillet; turn the pancake when bubbles appear on the surface and let it cook for 1 more minute or so.
4. Place 3 pancakes on a plate and drizzle with honey or fruit syrup.

Serving Suggestion:
Serve with fresh fruit.

Frittata with Asparagus, Tomato, and Fontina Cheese
Servers 4-6

6 large eggs
2 Tbsp. milk
½ tsp. salt, plus a pinch
¼ tsp. freshly ground black pepper
1 Tbsp. olive oil
12 oz. asparagus, trimmed, cut into ¼- to ½-inch pieces
1 tomato, seeded, diced
1 tsp. salt
3 oz. Fontina cheese, diced

1. Preheat the broiler. Whisk the eggs, milk, ½ teaspoon salt, and pepper in a medium bowl to blend; set aside.
2. Heat the oil in a 9 ½-inch-diameter nonstick ovenproof skillet over medium heat. Add the asparagus and sauté until crisp-tender, about 2 minutes. Raise the heat to medium-high. Add the tomato and pinch of salt, and sauté 2 minutes longer. Pour the egg mixture over the asparagus mixture and cook for a few minutes until the eggs start to set. Sprinkle with cheese. Reduce heat to medium-low and cook until the frittata is almost set but the top is still runny, about 2 minutes.
3. Place the skillet under the broiler. Broil until the top is set and golden brown, about 5 minutes.
4. Let the frittata stand 2 minutes. Using a rubber spatula, loosen the frittata from skillet and slide onto a plate.

Serving suggestion:
Crusty French bread slices with fruit spread and hash browns.

Fresh Muesli

Serves 4

3 cups rolled oats
2 cups coarse oat bran
½ cup almonds, sliced
½ cup whole almonds
½ cup pumpkin seeds
½ cup sunflower seeds
¾ cup dried unsweetened coconut
¼ cup currants
¼ cup dried cherries
¼ cup golden raisins
¼ cup dried mangoes, chopped
¼ cup dried apples, chopped
¼ cup dried apricots, chopped

1. Combine all the ingredients in a large bowl, and transfer to an airtight container to store.

    Serving Suggestion:
    Serve with milk and honey or over yogurt with a handful of berries.

Waffles

Serves 4

1 egg
1 ¼ cups low-fat milk
¼ cup canola oil
½ tsp. vanilla extract
1 ½ cups all-purpose flour
2 tsp. sugar
3 tsp. baking powder
¼ tsp. salt
Fresh honey or maple syrup

1. Preheat waffle iron. Beat eggs in large bowl with hand mixer until fluffy. Beat in milk, oil, and vanilla extract until well mixed.
2. Combine flour, sugar, baking powder, and salt. Slowly add to the wet ingredients, beating just until smooth.
3. Spray preheated waffle iron with nonstick cooking spray. Pour mix onto hot waffle iron. Cook until golden brown.
4. Place a waffle on a plate and drizzle with honey or maple syrup.

Serving Suggestion:
Serve with fresh fruit and milk.

CHAPTER 15
Tasty Lunches

Most individuals tend to skip lunch, in the hope of accomplishing more at the office or fitting in a few errands during the time they would be spending to eat a healthy meal. Taking a few simple steps to plan ahead and having a balanced and healthy lunch ready for on the go or at home will be of great benefit the body and how it will perform throughout the remainder of the day.

It is easy to get in a rut and have the same chicken salad or turkey sandwich every day, but some variety adds a lot in terms of both excitement and nutrition.

Try the following lunch ideas, a different one every day, to help give you the much needed energy to keep you going strong through the day.

Turkey Wrap

Serves 4

4 10-inch flour tortillas
4 tsp. low-fat mayo
4 tsp. Dijon-style mustard
8 oz. turkey breast, sliced
4 oz. low-fat cheddar cheese, shredded
2 cups romaine lettuce, shredded
1 tomato, chopped
Salt and pepper as desired

1. Spread each tortilla with 1 tsp. of mayo and mustard.
2. Top each with 2 oz. of turkey, 1 oz. of cheese, ½ cup lettuce, ¼ cup of tomatoes, and salt and pepper if desired.
3. Fold in the sides of the tortilla, roll it up burrito style, and cut it in half.
4. Place the wrap on a plate and serve.

Serving Suggestion:
Serve with carrot sticks and green tea.

The Famous PB&J Sandwich

Serves 4

8 slices whole wheat bread
8 Tbsp. peanut butter
4 Tbsp. fruit spread

1. Spread 4 of the 8 slices of bread with 2 Tbsp. of the peanut butter and 1 Tbsp. of the fruit spread.
2. Put the other 4 slices of bread on top and cut in half at an angle.
3. Place on a plate and serve.

Serving Suggestion:
Serve with apple slices and milk.

Bean Quesadillas

Serves 4

1 cup sliced onion
1 tsp. minced garlic
1 jalapeno, minced
1 tsp. ground cumin
15 oz. can black beans, drained
15 oz. can pinto beans, drained
1 cup chopped tomato
1 Tbsp. cilantro to taste
1 tsp. salt
½ tsp. pepper to taste
8 tortillas
1 ½ cups cheddar cheese, shredded
Salsa
Sour cream

1. Preheat oven to 450 degrees.
2. Spray skillet with cooking spray; heat over medium heat. Sauté onion, garlic, jalapeno, and cumin until crisp-tender, about 5 minutes.
3. Add beans to skillet and mix. Add tomato and cilantro to the skillet and stir, cooking for about 1-2 minutes.
4. Spoon a nice helping of the mixture onto each tortilla. Add the cheese. Fold over and spray both sides with cooking spray.
5. Bake on cookie sheet for about 5-7 minutes or until a little brown.
6. Place on a plate, cut into triangles, and serve with salsa and sour cream.

Serving Suggestion:
Serve with orange slices.

Harvest Spinach Salad

Serves 4

1 bunch spinach (about 12 cups)
½ cup dried cherries
½ cup dried apricot halves, cut into strips
3 scallions, thinly sliced
1 green apple, cored and thinly sliced
½ cup seedless red grapes, cut in half
¼ cup walnuts, coarsely chopped
2 tsp. apple cider vinegar
2 Tbsp. extra-virgin olive oil
1 tsp. salt
½ tsp. ground black pepper
2 cups feta cheese, crumbled

1. Combine spinach, cherries, apricots, scallions, apple slices, grapes, and walnuts in a large bowl.
2. Whisk together vinegar and olive oil; season to taste with salt and pepper.
3. Place the salad on plates and pour vinaigrette over it; add the cheese and serve.

Serving Suggestion:
Serve with French bread slices.

Spicy Chili Beans Over Rice

Serves 6

1 small onion, chopped
3 cloves garlic, minced
1 Tbsp. olive oil
1 14.5 oz. can pinto beans
1 14.5 oz. can kidney beans
1 14.5 oz. can black beans
1 14.5 oz. can diced tomatoes
1 4 oz. can green chilies, chopped
½ Tbsp. chili powder
¼ tsp. cumin
1 tsp. salt
½ tsp. pepper
1 ½ cups low-fat cheddar cheese, shredded
½ cup low-fat sour cream
¼ cup fresh parsley, chopped
3-4 cups cooked brown rice

1. Heat a large skillet over medium-high heat. Add olive oil, onion, and garlic. Cook until soft, about 5-7 minutes.
2. Add tomatoes, beans, chilies and spices; simmer 15-20 minutes.
3. Serve on a plate over cooked brown rice; top with cheese, sour cream and fresh parsley.

Serving Suggestion:
Serve with a cornbread muffin and a nice glass of sweet lemonade.

Tuna Pita Sandwich

Serves 4

2 6 ½ oz. cans tuna (in water), drained
½ cup carrots, shredded
1 celery stalk, diced
1 small onion, diced
¼ cup low-fat mayo
1 tsp. Dijon-style mustard
1 tsp. salt
½ tsp. pepper
8 pieces of leaf lettuce
8 slices of tomato
4 whole grain pitas, halved

1. In a large bowl combine tuna, carrots, celery, and onion; set aside.
2. In a small bowl stir together mayo, mustard, salt, and pepper.
3. Pour the dressing over the tuna mixture and stir until well coated.
4. Take the halved pitas and place 1 lettuce leaf and 1 slice of tomato in each one. Divide tuna mixture into 4 portions and fill each pita half.
5. Place on a plate and serve.

Serving Suggestion:
Serve with apple slices.

Roast Beef and Cheese Sandwich

Serves 4

8 slices whole wheat bread
4 tsp. low-fat mayo
4 tsp. Dijon-style mustard
8 oz. roast beef, sliced
4 oz. low-fat cheddar cheese, slices
4 leaves of romaine lettuce
8 slices of tomato
Salt and pepper as desired

1. Spread 4 of the 8 slices of bread with 1 tsp. mayo and 1 tsp. of mustard.
2. Layer with 1 lettuce leaf, 2 slices of tomato, 2 oz. of roast beef, and 1 oz. of cheese.
3. Put the other 4 slices of bread on top and cut in half.
4. Place on a plate and serve.

Serving Suggestion:
Serve with watermelon wedges.

CHAPTER 16
Easy and Delicious Dinners

Dinners do not have to become a thing of the past. There are so many versatile, quick, and easy meals out there just waiting to be tried. Finding time to prepare a balanced and healthy dinner just takes a little planning, a few ingredients, and a kitchen waiting to be used.

Try the following dinner ideas, a different one every day, and you will soon find the joy of cooking easy and delicious dinners.

Fettuccine Alfredo

Serves 4-6

1 16 oz. pkg. fettuccine
1 stick of butter
1 cup parmesan cheese, shredded
1 cup whipping cream
4 eggs
½ Tbsp. salt
2 Tbsp. fresh parsley, chopped

1. Cook pasta according to package directions; drain and set aside.
2. In a saucepan over medium heat, add the butter and let it melt completely.
3. Stir in the parmesan cheese until melted; pour in whipping cream and whisk all ingredients together until smooth.
4. Place eggs in a small bowl; beat slightly. Stir a small amount of hot cream mixture into eggs; stir. Pour eggs into the hot cream mixture in the saucepan.
5. Cook sauce over low heat, stirring constantly with a whisk until thoroughly heated, about 5 minutes.
6. Toss pasta with the cream sauce until well coated; add salt and parsley.
7. Place on plates and serve.

Serving Suggestion:
Serve with warm French bread and a crisp salad tossed with Italian dressing.

Grilled Tenderloin with Warm Vegetable Salad

Serves 4

4 4-oz. beef tenderloin steaks
½ tsp. salt, divided
½ tsp. black pepper, divided
1 tsp. mixed dried herb seasoning
2 small zucchini, halved lengthwise
2 small yellow squash, halved lengthwise
2 plum tomatoes, halved lengthwise
2 green onions
2 Tbsp. red wine vinegar
2 tsp. garlic, minced
Cooking spray

1. Prepare grill or broiler.
2. Sprinkle steaks with 1/4 tsp. salt and 1/4 tsp. pepper; set aside.
3. Combine 1/4 tsp. salt, 1/4 tsp. pepper, herb seasoning, zucchini, yellow squash, tomatoes, onions, red wine vinegar and garlic in a large zip-top plastic bag. Seal and shake to coat.
4. Place tenderloin steaks on grill rack or broiler pan coated with cooking spray; cook for 4 minutes on each side or until desired degree of doneness.
5. Place zucchini and yellow squash on grill rack or broiler pan coated with cooking spray; cook 3 minutes on each side or until tender. Place tomato and onions on grill rack or broiler pan; cook 2 minutes or just until tender.
6. Places steaks and grilled vegetables on plates and serve.

Serving Suggestion:
Serve with rice pilaf and orange slices.

Chunky Vegetarian Chili

Serves 4-6

1 Tbsp. canola oil
2 cups onion, chopped
½ cup yellow bell pepper, chopped
½ cup green bell pepper, chopped
2 garlic cloves, minced
1 Tbsp. brown sugar
1 ½ Tbsp. chili powder
1 tsp. ground cumin
1 tsp. dried oregano
1 tsp. salt
½ tsp. pepper
2 16-oz. cans stewed tomatoes, not drained
2 15-oz. cans black beans, rinsed and drained
1 15-oz. can kidney beans, rinsed and drained
1 15-oz. can pinto beans, rinsed and drained

1. Heat oil in a large saucepan over medium-high heat. Add onion, bell peppers, and garlic; sauté 5 minutes or until tender.
2. Add sugar and remaining ingredients and bring to a boil.
3. Reduce heat and simmer for 30 minutes.
4. Place in bowls and serve.

Serving Suggestions:
Serve with skillet cornbread and coleslaw.

Mostaccioli Pasta

Serves 4-6

1 lb. mostaccioli pasta
¼ cup olive oil
2 Tbsp. balsamic vinegar
3 cloves garlic
2 oz. fresh basil
1 tsp. salt
¼ tsp. pepper
2 cups ripe tomatoes, cubed
¾ cup kalamata olives, sliced

1. Heat water in a large pot; cook pasta according to the box directions; drain and set aside.
2. In a blender or food processor, combine olive oil, balsamic vinegar, and garlic until well mixed.
3. Add basil, salt, and pepper; mix for 1 minute or until well blended.
4. Pour sauce over warm pasta; add tomatoes and kalamata olives; toss well. Garnish with remaining basil leaves.
5. Place on plates and serve.

Serving Suggestion:
Serve with freshly baked knot rolls and a tossed salad with a balsamic and herb dressing.

Grilled Chicken Breasts with Sun-Dried Tomato Pesto
Serves 4

4 4-oz. skinless chicken breasts
¼ cup balsamic vinegar
½ cup fresh basil leaves, plus a few for garnish
2 Tbsp. olive oil
2 tsp. salt
½ tsp. black pepper
12 sun-dried tomatoes, in olive oil
1 Tbsp. pine nuts
1 clove garlic
1 Tbsp. Parmesan cheese, freshly grated
3 Tbsp. chicken broth

1. In a large zip-top bag, combine balsamic vinegar, ¼ cup of basil leaves, 1 Tbsp. olive oil, 1 tsp. salt, and ¼ tsp. pepper. Add chicken breasts and seal the bag. Turn it over a few times until chicken is evenly coated. (This can be done a day in advance and stored in the refrigerator.)
2. For the sun-dried tomato pesto, combine sun-dried tomatoes, pine nuts, garlic, and the remaining ¼ cup basil leaves in a food processor. Process until the mixture is finely ground. Add the Parmesan cheese, the remaining olive oil, chicken broth, 1 tsp. salt, and ¼ tsp. Pepper; process for a few more seconds to combine.
3. Preheat oven on broil to medium-high.
4. Place chicken on broiling pan and grill on each side until cooked thoroughly, about 6 minutes per side.
5. Top each chicken breast with a dollop of sun-dried tomato pesto and garnish with basil leaves.
6. Place chicken on a plate and serve.

Serving Suggestion:
Serve with couscous and sautéed zucchini and yellow squash.

Spinach Quiche

Serves 4-6

1 9-inch basic pie crust (purchased is fine)
2 cups cheddar cheese, shredded
2 Tbsp. flour
1 10 oz. pkg. frozen spinach, cooked, well drained
1 Tbsp. olive oil
1 clove garlic, diced
1 small onion, chopped
1 cup milk
2 eggs, lightly beaten
1 tsp. salt
½ tsp. pepper

1. Preheat oven to 350 degrees.
2. Mix cheese with flour in medium bowl; set aside.
3. In a skillet, sauté garlic, onion, and spinach until tender and hot.
4. Add spinach, milk, eggs, salt and pepper to cheese mixture; mix well.
5. Pour into pie crust and bake for 1 hour or until set.
6. Remove from oven and let cool for 10-15 minutes.
7. Place on a plate and serve.

Serving Suggestion:
Serve with a tossed baby greens salad with Italian dressing and hash browns.

Grilled Salmon Sandwich

Serves 4

4 6-oz. salmon fillets
3 Tbsp. dry mustard
4 Tbsp. packed light-brown sugar
1 tsp. soy sauce
2 Tbsp. olive oil
1 tsp. salt
½ tsp. pepper
4 cups arugula leaves, slightly wet
8 slices tomato
6 slices sourdough bread, toasted lightly

1. Combine mustard and sugar in a small bowl. Stir in 1 ½ Tbsp. water. Add soy sauce and 1 tsp. oil. Set aside.
2. Heat a grill or grill pan until very hot. Brush salmon with remaining oil; season with salt and pepper. Grill for 5 minutes, or until browned. Turn and grill for another 5 minutes, or to desired doneness.
3. Toast bread; layer 4 of the toasted sourdough slices each with wilted arugula, tomato slices, and a salmon fillet. Drizzle remaining mustard sauce on salmon. Top with the other 4 slices of sourdough bread.
4. Place salmon sandwiches on a plate and serve.

Serving Suggestion:
Serve with seasoned potato wedges and ice tea.

CHAPTER 17
Pick-me-up Snacks

Snacks are what fill the gaps between meals, and snacks are necessary to keep the body's blood sugar level and energy constant during the day. It is best to have a snack about 3-4 hours after a main meal.

Breakfast —> Midmorning Snack
Lunch —> Midday Snack
Dinner —> Evening Snack

When most individuals think of snacks, they picture potato chips, candy bars, and sodas. These forms of snacks are empty calories. They provide high amounts of calories, fat, sugar, and salt, but little or no nutrients, vitamins, and minerals that the body is designed to use.

A healthy snack provides the body with needed nutrition and will keep the blood sugar level from dropping too low, which leaves the body sluggish and craving sweets. Eating a healthy snack in between meals will keep the metabolism efficient, and such a snack will not load the body down with unwanted calories, fat, sugar, and salt.

Choose snacks with a lot of pick-me-up power of energy-giving carbohydrates, proteins, and fats. Keep these snacks available wherever you are—at the office, in the car, in your briefcase or backpack, even in your purse. When you have good choices of healthy snacks available, you are not as likely to turn to an unhealthy snack to get you to the next meal.

Try the following snack ideas, and you will soon find that snacks can be healthy and tasty at the same time. Samples of some healthy snacks are as follows:

- 1 apple with 1 low-fat cheese stick

- 1 whole grain bagel with 2 oz. low-fat cream cheese

- ¼ cup trail mix and dried fruit

- Protein drink/smoothie

- 1 8 oz. low-fat fruit yogurt with ½ cup granola

- ¾ cup cottage cheese with ½ cup pineapple chunks

- 2 granola bars with 2 Tbsp. peanut butter

- 2 oz. lean meat with 5-6 whole grain crackers

- 1 low-fat raisin bran muffin with 1 cup low-fat milk

Carrot Raisin Bars

Serves 16

3 Tbsp. butter
½ cup brown sugar
1 egg white
1 tsp. vanilla extract
¾ cup whole wheat flour
¾ cup quick-cooking oats
¼ cup wheat germ
1 tsp. ground cinnamon
1 tsp. baking powder
1 ¼ cups grated carrots (about 2 1/2 medium)
½ cup golden raisins

1. Preheat oven to 350 degrees.
2. Combine butter and brown sugar in food processor or mixer and process until smooth. Add egg white and vanilla extract and process until smooth.   .
3. In a bowl, combine flour, oats, wheat germ, cinnamon, and baking powder. Add flour mixture to butter mixture and process to mix well. Fold in carrots and raisins.
4. Coat an 8-inch square pan with nonstick spray. Pat mixture evenly into pan. Bake for 25-30 minutes or until a toothpick comes out clean. Cool to room temperature and cut into 16 squares.

Peanut Butter Energy Balls

Serves 30

1 cup peanut butter
1 cup honey
2 cups instant milk
1 tsp. vanilla extract
1 cup wheat germ

1. In a large bowl, mix together all the ingredients, except wheat germ. Place wheat germ in a separate bowl.
2. Form mixture into 1-inch balls and roll in wheat germ until lightly coated.
3. Store in an airtight container and refrigerate for up to a week.

Low-Fat Raisin Bran Muffins

Serves 12

1 ½ cups wheat bran
½ cup all-purpose flour
½ cup whole wheat flour
¾ cup brown sugar
1 tsp. baking soda
1 tsp. baking powder
1 tsp. cinnamon
½ tsp. salt
1 cup raisins
½ cup unsweetened applesauce
½ tsp. vanilla extract
1 egg
1 cup low-fat buttermilk

1. Preheat oven to 375 degrees. Grease muffin pan or use paper muffin cups.
2. In a large bowl, mix together wheat bran, all-purpose flour, whole wheat flour, brown sugar, baking soda, baking powder, cinnamon, salt, and raisins. Set aside.
3. In a smaller bowl, mix together unsweetened applesauce, vanilla extract, egg and milk.
4. Combine wet ingredients with dry ingredients and mix until just blended.
5. Divide batter evenly into the muffin pan/cups. Bake for 15–20 minutes, or until tops spring back when touched lightly.

Strawberry Smoothie

Serves 4

2 scoops vanilla protein powder
½ Tbsp. wheat germ
1 Tbsp. honey
1 cup low-fat milk
1 ½ cups low-fat vanilla ice cream
1 cup fresh strawberries

1. In a blender, combine all ingredients and blend until smooth or to desired consistency.

Trail Mix

Serves 15

1 cup raw peanuts
1 cup raw almonds
1 cup raw walnuts
1 cup raw pumpkin seeds
1 cup raw sunflower seeds
2 cups raisins

1. In a large bowl, combine all the ingredients until well mixed.
2. Measure out ¼ cup servings and store in individual zip-top bags.

GLOSSARY

-A-

Absorption: the passage of nutrients from the GI tract into either the blood or the lymph.

Acetyl CoA (ASS-eh-teel or ah-SEET-il, coh-AY): a 2-carbon compound to which a molecule of CoA is attached.

Acid-Base Balance: the equilibrium in the body between acid and base concentrations.

Acidosis: above-normal acidity in the blood and body fluids.

Acids: compounds that release hydrogen ions in a solution.

Additives: substances not normally consumed as foods but added to food either intentionally or by accident.

Adequate Intake (AI): the average amount of a nutrient that appears sufficient to maintain a specified criterion; a value used as a guide for nutrient intake when an RDA cannot be determined.

Adipose (DD-ih-poce) Tissue: the body's fat tissue; consists of masses of fat-storing cells.

Adolescence: the period from the beginning of puberty until maturity.

Adrenal Glands: glands adjacent to, and just above, each kidney.

Alcohol: a class of organic compounds containing hydroxyl (OH) groups.

Aldosterone (al-DOS-ter-own): a hormone secreted by the adrenal glands that stimulates the reabsorption of sodium by the kidneys, thereby regulating chloride and potassium concentrations, blood volume, and blood pressure.

Amino (a-MEEN-oh) Acids: building blocks of proteins. Each contains an amino group, an acid group, a hydrogen atom, and a distinctive side group, all attached to a central carbon atom.

Amino Acid Pool: the supply of amino acids derived from either food proteins or body proteins that collect in the cells and circulating blood and stand ready to be incorporated in proteins and other compounds or used for energy.

Amylase (AM-ih-lace): an enzyme that hydrolyzes amylose (a form of starch). Amylase is a carbohydrase, an enzyme that breaks down carbohydrates.

Anabolism (an-ABB-o-lism): reactions in which small molecules are put together to build larger ones. Anabolic reactions require energy.

Anemia (ah-NEE-me-ah): literally, "too little blood." Anemia is any condition in which too few red blood cells are present, or the red blood cells are immature (and therefore large) or too small or contain too little hemoglobin to carry the normal amount of oxygen to the tissue. It is not a disease itself, but can be a symptom of many different disease conditions.

Anorexia (an-oh-RECK-see-ah) Nervosa: an eating disorder characterized by a refusal to maintain a minimally normal body weight and a distortion in perception of body shape and weight.

Antibodies: large proteins of the blood and body fluids, produced by the immune system in response to the invasion of the body by foreign molecules (usually proteins called antigens). Antibodies combine with and inactivate the foreign invaders, thus protecting the body.

Antidiuretic Hormone (ADH): a hormone released by the pituitary gland in response to highly concentrated blood. The kidneys respond by reabsorbing water, thus preventing water loss.

Antigens: substances that elicit the formation of antibodies or an inflammation reaction from the immune system. A bacterium, a virus, a toxin, and a protein in food that causes allergy are all examples of antigens.

Antioxidants: compounds that protect others from oxidation by being oxidized themselves; preservaties that prevent rancidity of fats in foods and other damage to food caused by oxygen.

Appetite: the integrated response to the sight, smell, thought, or taste of food that initiates or delays eating.

Arteries: vessels that carry blood away from the heart.

Arthritis: inflammation of a joint, usually accompanied by pain, swelling, and structural changes.

Atoms: the smallest components of an element that have all of the properties of the element.

ATP or Adenosine (ah-DEN-oh-seen) Triphosphate (try-FOS-fate): a common high-energy compound composed of a purine (adenine), a sugar (ribose), and three phosphate groups.

-B-

Balance (dietary): providing foods of a number of types in proportion to each other, such that foods rich in some nutrients do not crowd out of the diet foods that are rich in other nutrients.

Basal Metabolic Rate (BMR): the rate of energy used for metabolism under specified conditions. For example, after a 12-hour fast and restful sleep, or without any physical activity, or emotional excitement, and in a comfortable setting.

Basal Metabolism: the energy needed to maintain life when a body is at complete digestive, physical, and emotional rest.

Beta-carotene (Bay-tah KARE-oh-teen): one of the carotenoids; an orange pigment and vitamin A precursor found in plants. A **precursor** is a compound that can be converted into an active vitamin.

Bile: an emulsifier that prepares fats and oils for digestion; an exocrine secretion made by the liver, stored in the gallbladder, and released into the small intestine when needed.

Binders: chemical compounds in foods that combine with nutrients (especially minerals) to form complexes the body cannot absorb.

Bioavailability: the rate at and the extent to which a nutrient is absorbed and used.

Biotin (BY-oh-tin): a B vitamin that functions as a coenzyme in metabolism.

Body Composition: the proportions of muscle, bone, fat, and other tissue that make up a person's total body weight.

Body Mass Index (BMI): an index of a person's weight in relation to height; determined by dividing the weight (in kilograms) by the square of the height (in meters).

Branched-chain Amino Acids: the amino acids leucine, isoleucine, and valine, which are present in large amounts in skeletal muscle tissue; falsely promoted as fuel for exercising muscles.

Bulimia (byoo-LEEM-ee-ah) Nervosa: an eating disorder characterized by repeated episodes of binge eating usually followed by self-induced vomiting, misuse of laxatives or diuretics, fasting, or excessive exercise.

-C-

Caffeine: a natural stimulant found in many common foods and beverages, including coffee, tea, and chocolate; may enhance endurance by stimulating fatty acid release but also causes fluid losses. High doses cause headaches, trembling, rapid heart, and other undesirable side effects.

Calcium: the most abundant mineral in the body; found primarily in the body's bones and teeth.

Calories: units by which energy is measured in **kilocalories** (1000 calories equal 1 kilocalorie), abbreviated **kcalories** or **kcal**. A capitalized version is also sometimes used: **Calories**. One kcalorie is the amount of heat necessary to raise the temperature of 1 kilogram (kg) of water 1°C.

Cancer: diseases that result from the unchecked growth of malignant tumors.

Capillaries (CAP-ill-aries): small vessels that branch from an artery. Capillaries connect arteries to veins. Exchange of oxygen, nutrients, and waste materials take place across capillary walls.

Carbohydrates: compounds composed of carbon, oxygen, and hydrogen arranged as monosaccharides or multiples of monosaccharides. Most, but not all, carbohydrates have a ratio of one carbon molecule to one water molecule.

Cardiovascular Disease (CVD): a general term for all diseases of the heart and blood vessels. Atherosclerosis is the main cause of CVD. When the arteries that carry blood to the heart muscle become blocked, the heart suffers damage known as **coronary heart disease (CHD)**.

Carotenoids (kah-ROT-eh-noyds): pigments commonly found in plants and animals, some of which have vitamin A activity. The carotenoids with greatest vitamin A activity is **beta-carotene**.

Catabolism (ca-TAB-o-lism): reactions in which larger molecules are broken down to smaller ones. Catabolic reactions usually release energy.

Catalyst (CAT-uh-list): a compound that facilitates chemical reactions without itself being changed in the process.

Cell: the basic unit of life, of which all living things are composed. Every cell is surrounded by a membrane and contains cytoplasm, within which are organelles and a nucleus; the cell nucleus contains chromosomes.

Cell Membrane: the membrane that surrounds the cell and encloses its contents; made primarily of lipid and protein.

Chlorophyll (KLO-row-fil): the green pigment of plants, which absorbs light and transfers the energy to other molecules, thereby initiating photosynthesis.

Cholesterol (koh-LESS-ter-ol): one of the sterols containing four carbon rings and a carbon side chain.

Choline (KOH-leen): a nitrogen-containing compound found in foods and made in the body from the amino acid methionine. Choline is part of the phospholipids lecithin and the neurotransmitter acetylcholine.

Chromium (CROW-mee-um): a trace mineral supplement; falsely promoted as building muscle enhancing energy, and burning fat. Picolinate (pick-oh-LYN-ate) is a derivative of the amino acid tryptophan that seems to enhance chromium absorption.

Chromosome: a set of structures within the nucleus of every cell that contains the cell's genetic material, DNA, associated with other materials (primarily proteins).

Chronic Diseases: long-duration degenerative diseases characterized by deterioration of the body organs. Examples include heart disease, cancer, and diabetes.

Chyme (KIME): the semiliquid mass of partly digested food expelled by the stomach into the duodenum.

CoA (coh-AY): coenzyme A; the coenzyme derived from the B vitamin pantothenic acid and central to energy metabolism.

Collagen (KOL-ah-jen): the protein from which connective tissues such as scars, tendons, ligaments, and the foundations of bones and teeth are made.

Complementary Proteins: two or more proteins whose amino acid assortments complement each other in such a way that the essential amino acids missing from one are supplied by the other.

Complete Protein: a dietary protein containing all the essential amino acids in relatively the same amounts that human beings require. It may also contain nonessential amino acids.

Complex Carbohydrates (**starches** and **fibers**): polysaccharides composed of straight or branched chains of monosaccharides.

Compound: a substance composed of two or more different atoms—for example, water.

Conception: the union of the male sperm and the female ovum; fertilization.

Constipation: the condition of having infrequent or difficult bowel movements.

Coronary Heart Disease (CHD): the damage that occurs when the blood vessels carrying blood to the heart (the coronary arteries) become narrow and occluded.

-D-

Daily Values (DV): reference values developed by the FDA specifically for use on food labels.

Deamination (dee-AM-eh_NAY-shun): removal of the amino (NH2) group from a compound such as amino acid.

Deficient: the amount of a nutrient below which almost all healthy people can be expected, over time, to experience deficiency symptoms.

Dehydration: the condition in which body water losses exceed water intake. Symptoms include thirst, dry skin and mucous membranes, rapid heartbeat, low blood pressure, and weakness.

DHEA (Dehydroepiandrosterone) and **Androstenedione**: hormones made in the adrenal glands that serve as precursors to the male hormone testosterone.

Diabetes (DYE-uh-BEET-eez) **Mellitus** (MELL-ih-tus or mell-EYE-tus): a metabolic disorder of carbohydrate metabolism characterized by altered glucose regulation and utilization, usually resulting from insufficient or ineffective insulin.

Diarrhea: the frequent passage of watery bowel movements.

Diet: the foods and beverages a person eats and drinks.

Dietary Reference Intakes (DRI): a set of values for the dietary nutrient intakes of healthy people in the United States and Canada. These values are used for planning and assessing diets and include:
- Estimated Average Requirements.
- Recommended Dietary Allowances.
- Adequate Intakes.
- Tolerable Upper Intake Levels.

Digestion: the process by which food is broken down into absorbable units.

Digestive Enzymes: proteins found in digestive juices that act on food substances, causing them to break down into simpler compounds.

Digestive System: all the organs and glands associated with the ingestion and digestion of food.

Dipeptide (dye-PEP-tide): two amino acids bonded together.

Disaccharides (dye-SACK-uh-rides): pairs of monosaccharides linked together.

Distilled Water: water that has been vaporized and recondensed, leaving it free of dissolved minerals.

Drug: a substance that can modify one or more of the body's functions.

Duodenum (doo-oh-DEEN-um, doo-ODD-num): the top portion of the small intestine.

-E-

Eating Disorders: disturbances in eating behavior that jeopardize a person's physical or psychological health.

Edema (eh-DEEM-uh): the swelling of body tissue caused by excessive amounts of fluid in the interstitial spaces; seen in protein deficiency (among other conditions).

Electrolytes: salts that dissolve in water and dissociate into charged particles called ions.

Electron Transport Chain (ETC): the final pathway in energy metabolism where the electrons from hydrogen are passed to oxygen and the energy released is trapped in the bonds of APT.

Element: a substance composed of atoms that are alike.

Embryo (EM-bree-oh): the developing infant from two to eight weeks after conception.

Emulsifier (ee-MUL-sih-fire): a substance with both water-soluble and fat-soluble portions that promotes the mixing of oils and fats in a watery solution.

Energy: the capacity to do work. The energy in food is chemical energy. The body can convert this chemical energy to mechanical, electrical, or heat energy.

Energy-Yielding Nutrients: the nutrients that break down to yield energy the body can use:
- Carbohydrate.
- Protein.
- Fat.

Enriched: the addition to a food of nutrients that were lost during processing so that the food will meet a specified standard.

Enzymes: proteins that facilitate chemical reactions without being changed in the process; protein catalysts.

Epinephrine (EP-ih-NEFF-rin): a hormone of the adrenal glad that modulates the stress response; formerly called **adrenaline**.

Esophagus (ee-SOFF-ah-gus): the food pipe; the conduit from the mouth to the stomach.

Essential Amino Acids: amino acids that the body cannot synthesize in amounts sufficient to meet physiological needs.

Essential Fatty Acids: fatty acids needed by the body, but not made by it in amounts sufficient to meet physiological needs.

Essential Nutrients: nutrients a person must obtain from food because the body cannot make them for itself in sufficient quantity to meet physiological needs; also called **indispensable nutrients**. About 40 nutrients are known to be essential for human beings.

Estimated Average Requirement: the amount of a nutrient that will maintain a specific biochemical or physiological function in half the people of a given age and gender group.

-F-

Fats: lipids in foods or the body; composed mostly of triglycerides.

Fatty Acids: an organic compound composed of a carbon chain with hydrogens attached and an acid group (COOH) at one end.

Fatty Acid Oxidation: the metabolic breakdown of fatty acids to acetyl CoA; also called **beta oxidation**.

FDA (Food and Drug Administration): a part of the Department of Health and Human Services' Public Health Service that is responsible for ensuring the safety and wholeness of all foods processed and sold in interstate commerce except meat, poultry, and eggs (which are under the jurisdiction of the USDA); inspecting food plants and important foods; and setting standards for food composition.

Ferment: to digest in the absence of oxygen.

Fetus (FEET-us): the developing infant from eight weeks after conception until term.

Fibers: in plant foods, the *nonstarch polysaccharides* that are not digested by human digestive enzymes, although some are digested by GI tract bacteria. Fibers include cellulose, hemicelluloses, pectins, gums, and mucilages and the non-polysaccharides lignins, cutins, and tannins.

Fluid Balance: maintenance of the proper types and amounts of fluid in each compartment of the body fluids.

Folate (FOLE-ate): a B vitamin; also known as folic acid, folacin, or pteroyglutamic (tare-o-EEL-glue-TAM-ick) acid PGA). The coenzyme forms are DHF (dihydrofolate) and THF (tetrahydrofolate).

Follicle-Stimulating Hormone (FSH): a hormone that stimulates maturation of the ovarian follicles in the females and the production of sperm in males. (The ovarian follicles are part of the female reproductive system where the eggs are produced.)

Food Intolerances: adverse reactions to foods that do not involve the immune system.

Foods: products derived from plants or animals that can be taken into the body to yield energy and nutrients for the maintenance of life and the growth and repair of tissues.

Fortified: the addition to a food of nutrients that were either not originally present or present in insignificant amounts. Fortification can be used to correct or prevent a widespread nutrient deficiency or to balance the total nutrient profile of a food.

Free Radicals: unstable and highly reactive atoms or molecules that have one or more unpaired electrons in the outer orbital.

Fructose (FRUK-tose or FROOK-tose): a monosaccharide. Sometimes known as fruit sugar or **levulose**, fructose is found abundantly in fruits, honey, and saps.

Fuel: compounds that cells can use for energy. The major fuels include glucose, fatty acids, and amino acids; other fuels include ketone bodies, lactic acid, glycerol, and alcohol.

-G-

Galactose (ga-LAK-tose): a monosaccharide; part of the disaccharide lactose.

Gallbladder: the organ that stores and concentrates bile. When it receives the signal that fat is present in the duodenum, the gallbladder contracts and squirts bile through the bile duct into the duodenum.

Gastric Glands: exocrine glands in the stomach wall that secrete gastric juice into the stomach.

Gastric Juice: the digestive secretion of the gastric glands of the stomach.

Gastrointestinal (GI) Tract: the digestive tract. The principal organs are the stomach and intestines.

Gestation(jes-TAY-shun): the period from conception to birth. For human beings, gestation last from 38 to 42 weeks. Pregnancy is often divided into thirds, called **trimesters**.

Gestational Diabetes: abnormal glucose tolerance that is first detected during pregnancy.

Gland: a cell or group of cells that secretes materials for special uses in the body. Glands may be **exocrine** (EKS-oh-crin) **glands**, secreting their materials "out" (into the digestive tract or onto the surface of the skin), or **endocrine** (EN-doe-crin) **glands**, secreting their materials "in" (into the blood).

Glucagon (GLOO-ka-gon): a hormone that is secreted by special cells in the pancreas in response to low blood glucose concentration and elicits release of glucose from storage.

Glucose (GLOO-kose): a monosaccharide; sometimes known as blood sugar or **dextrose**.

Glycerol (GLISS-er-ol); an alcohol composed of a three-carbon chain, which can serve as the backbone for a triglyceride.

Glycogen (GLY-co-gen): an animal polysaccharide composed of glucose; manufactured and stored in the liver and muscles as a storage form of glucose. Glycogen is not a significant food source of carbohydrate and is not counted as one of the complex carbohydrates in foods.

Glycolysis (gligh-COLL-ih-sis): the metabolic breakdown of glucose to pyruvate. Glycolysis does not require oxygen (anaerobic).

Growth Hormone (GH): a hormone secreted by the pituitary that regulates the cell division and protein synthesis needed for normal growth.

-H-

HDL (High-Density Lipoprotein): the type of lipoprotein that transports cholesterol back to the liver from the cells; composed primarily of protein.

Heart Attack: sudden tissue death caused by blockages of vessels that feed the heart muscle; also called **myocardial** (my-oh-KAR-dee-al) **infarction** (in-FARK-shun) or **cardiac arrest**.

Heartburn: a burning sensation in the chest area caused by backflow of the stomach acid into the esophagus.

Hemoglobin (HE-moh-GLOW-bin): the globular protein of the red blood cells that carries oxygen from the lungs to the cells throughout the body.

Hemorrhoids (HEM-oh-royds): painful swelling of the veins surrounding the rectum.

High-Quality Protein: an easily digestible, complete protein.

Histamine (HISS-tah-mean or HISS-tah-men): a substance produced by cells of the immune system as part of a local immune reaction to an antigen; participates in causing inflammation.

Homeostasis (HOME-ee-oh-STAY-sis): the maintenance of constant internal conditions (such as blood chemistry, temperature, and blood pressure) by the body's control systems. A homeostatic system is constantly reacting to external forces so as to maintain limits set by the body's needs.

Hormone: a chemical messenger. Hormones are secreted by variety of endocrine glands in response to altered conditions in the body. Each hormone travels to one or more specific target tissues or organs, where it elicits a specific response to maintain homeostasis.

Hydrochloric Acid: an acid composed of hydrogen and chloride atoms (HC1). The gastric glands normally produce this acid.

Hydrogenation (high-dro-gen-AY-shun): a chemical process by which hydrgens are added to monounsaturated or polyunsaturated fats to reduce the number of double bonds, making the fats more saturated (solid) and more resistant to the oxidation (protecting against rancidity). Hydrogenation produces *trans*-fatty acids.

Hydrolysis (high-DROL-ih-sis): a chemical reaction in which a major reaction is split into two products, with the addition of a hydrogen atom to one end and a hydroxyl group to the other (from water).

Hydrophilic (high-dro-FIL-ick): a term referring to water-loving, or water-soluble, substances.

Hydrophobic (high-dro-FOE-bick): a term referring to water-fearing, or non-water-soluble, substances; also known as **lipophilic** (fat loving).

Hypertension: higher-than-normal blood pressure. Hypertension that develops without an identifiable cause is known as *essential* or *primary hypertension*; hypertension that is caused by a specific disorder such as kidney disease is known as *secondary hypertension*.

-I-

Immune System: the body's natural defense system against foreign materials that have penetrated the skin or mucous membranes.

Immunity: the body's ability to recognize and eliminate foreign invaders.

Inorganic: not containing carbon or pertaining to living things.

Insoluble Fibers: indigestible food components that do not dissolve in water. Examples include the tough, fibrous structures found in the strings of celery and the skins of corn kernels.

Insulin (IN-suh-lin): a hormone secreted by special cells in the pancreas in response to (among other things) increased blood glucose concentration. The primary role of insulin is to control the transport of glucose from the bloodstream into the muscle and fat cells.

Insulin Resistance: the condition in which a normal amount of insulin produces a subnormal effect; a metabolic consequence of obesity.

Interstitial (IN-ter-STISH-al) **Fluid**: fluid between the cells, usually high inn sodium and chloride. Interstitial fluid is a large component of **extracellular fluid** (fluid outside the cells), which also includes plasma and the water of structures such as the skin and bones. Extracellular fluid accounts for approximately one-third of the body's water.

Ions (EYE-uns): atoms or molecules that have gained or lost electrons and therefore have electrical charges. Examples include the positively charged sodium ion and the negatively charged chloride ion.

Iron Deficiency: the state of having depleted iron stores.

Iron-Deficiency Anemia: Severe depletion of iron stores that results in low hemoglobin and small, pale, red blood cells.

-K-

Ketone (KEE-tone) **Bodies**: the product of the incomplete breakdown of fat when glucose is not available in the cells.

Ketosis (kee-TOE-sis): an undesirably high concentration of ketone bodies in the blood and urine.

-L-

Lactase: an enzyme that hydrolyzes lactose.

Lactation: production and secretion of breast milk for the purpose of nourishing and infant.

Lactic Acid: lactate, a 3-carbon compound produced from pyruvate during anaerobic metabolism.

Lactose (LAK-tose): a disaccharide composed of glucose and galactose; commonly known as milk sugar.

Large Intestine or Colon (COAL-un): the lower portion of intestine that completes the digestive process. Its segments are the ascending colon, the transverse colon, the descending colon, and the sigmoid colon.

LDL (Low-Density Lipoprotein): the type of lipoprotein derived from very-low-density lipoproteins (VLDL) as cells remove triglycerides from them; composed primarily of cholesterol.

Lecithin (LESS-uh-thin): one of the phospholipids; a compound of glycerol to which are attached two fatty acids, a phosphate group, and a choline molecule. Both nature and food industry use lecithin as an emulsifier to combine two ingredients that do not ordinarily mix, such as water and oil.

Legumes (lay-GYOOMS or LEG-yooms): plants of the bean and pea family, rich in high-quality protein compared with other plant-derived foods.

Linoleic (lin-oh-LAY-ick) Acid: an essential fatty acid with 18 carbons and two double bonds.

Linolenic (lin-oh-LEN-ick) Acid: an essential fatty acid with 18 carbons and three double bonds.

Lipase (LYE-pase): an enzyme that hydrolyzes lipids (fats).

Lipids: a family of compounds that includes triglycerides (fats and oils), phospholipids, and sterols.

Lipoprotein Lipase (LPL): an enzyme mounted on the surface of fat cells (and other cells) that hydrolyzes triglycerides passing by in the bloodstream and directs their parts into the cells, where they can be metabolized or reassembled for storage.

Lipoproteins (LIP-oh-PRO-teenz): clusters of lipids associated with proteins that serve as transport vehicles for lipids in the lymph and blood.

Liver: the organ that manufactures bile.

Luteinizing (LOO-tee-in-EYE-zing) **Hormone** (**LH**): a hormone that stimulates ovulation and the development of the corpus luteum (the small tissue that develops from a ruptured ovarian follicle and secretes hormones); so called because the follicle turns yellow as it matures. In men, LH stimulates testosterone secretion.

Lymph (LIMF): a clear yellowish fluid that is almost identical to blood except that it contains no red blood cells or platelets. Lymph from the GI tract transports fat and fat-soluble vitamins to the bloodstream via lymphatic vessels.

Lymphatic (lim-FAT-ic) **System**: a loosely organized system of vessels and ducts that convey fluids toward the heart. The GI part of the lymphatic system carries the products of digestion into the bloodstream.

Lymphocytes (LIM-foh-sites): white blood cells that participate in acquired immunity; B-cells and T-cells.

-M-

Magnesium: a cation with the body's cells, active in many enzyme systems.

Major Minerals: essential mineral nutrients found in the human body in amounts larger than 5 g; sometimes called **macrominerals**.

Malnutrition: any condition caused by excess or deficient food energy or nutrient intake or by an imbalance of nutrients.

Maltase: an enzyme that hydrolyzes maltose.

Maltose (MAWL-tose); a disaccharide composed of two glucose units; sometimes known as malt sugar.

Mammary Glands: glands of the female breast that secrete milk.

Matrix (MAY-tricks): the basic substance that gives form to a developing structure; in the body, the formative cells from which teeth and bones grow.

Matter: anything that takes up space and has mass.

Metabolism: the sum total of all the chemical reactions that go on in living cells. **Energy metabolism** includes all the reactions by which the body obtains and spends the energy from food.

Micelles (MY-cells): tiny spherical complexes of emulsified fat that arise during digestion. Each carries dozens of molecules of bile and fatty acids and/or monoglycerides.

Microvilli (MY-cro-VILL-ee or MY-cro-VILL-eye): tiny, hairlike projections on each cell of every villus that can trap nutrient particles and transport them into the cells.

Mineral Water: water from a spring or well that typically contains 250 to 500 ppm (parts per million) of minerals. Minerals give water a distinctive flavor.

Minerals: inorganic elements. Some minerals are essential nutrients required in small amounts.

Mitochondria (my-toh-KON-dree-uh); singular **mitochondrion**: the cellular organelles responsible for producing ATP aerobically; made of membranes (lipid and protein) with enzymes mounted on them.

Molecule: two or more atoms of the same or different elements joined by chemical bonds.

Molybdenum (mo-LIB-duh-num): a trace mineral.

Monoglycerides: molecules of glycerol with one fatty acid attached. A molecule of glycerol with two fatty acids attached is a **diglyceride**.

Monosaccharide (mon-oh-SACK-uh-ride): a carbohydrate form.

Monounsaturated Fatty Acid: a fatty acid that lacks two hydrogen atoms and has one double bond between carbons.

Mouth: the oral cavity containing the tongue and teeth.

Mucous (MYOO-kus): a slippery substance secreted by goblet cells of the GI lining (and other body linings) that protects the cells from exposure to digestive juices (and other destructive agents).

-N-

Net Protein Utilization (NPU): the amount of protein nitrogen that is retained from a given amount of protein nitrogen eaten; a measure of protein quality.

Niacin (NIGH-a-sin): a B vitamin.

Nitrogen Balance: the amount of nitrogen consumed as compared with the amount of the nitrogen excreted in a given period of time.

Nonessential Amino Acids: amino acids that the body can synthesize.

Nucleus: a major membrane-enclosed body within every cell, which contains the cell's genetic material, DNA, embedded in chromosomes.

Nutrient Additives: vitamins and minerals added to improve the nutrient value of foods.

Nutrient Density: a measure of the nutrients a food provides relative to the energy it provides. The more nutrients and the fewer calories, the higher the nutrient density.

Nutrients: chemical substances obtained from food and used in the body to provide energy, structural materials, and regulating agents to support growth, maintenance, and repair of the body's tissues. Nutrients may also reduce the risk of some diseases.

Nutritionist: a person who specializes in the study of nutrition.

-O-

Oils: liquid fats (at room temperature).

Omega: the last letter of the Greek alphabet, used by chemists to refer to the position of the first double bond from the methyl end in the fatty acid.

Omega-3 Fatty Acid: a polyunsaturated fatty acid in which the first double bond is three carbons away from the methyl end of the carbon chain.

Organic: a substance or molecule containing carbon-carbon bonds or carbon-hydrogen bonds. Some farmers call their produce "organic" because it is grown without manufactured fertilizers and pesticides, but by the definition given here, all foods are organic.

Osteoporosis (OS-tee-oh-pore-OH-sis): a condition of older persons in which the bones become porous and fragile due to a loss of minerals; also called **adult bone loss**.

Overweight: body weight above some standard of acceptable weight that is usually defined in relation to height (such as BMI).

Oxidants (OK-see-dants): compounds (such as oxygen itself) that oxidize other compounds. Compounds that prevent oxidation are called *anti*oxidants, whereas those that promote it are called *pro*oxidants.

Oxidation (OKS-ee-day-shun): the process of a substance combing with oxygen.

-P-

Pancreas: a gland that secrets digestive enzymes and juices into the duodenum.

Pancreatic (pank-ree-AT-ic) **Juice**: the exocrine secretion of the pancreas, containing enzymes for the digestion of carbohydrate, protein, and fat as well as bicarbonate, a neutralizing agent. The juice flows from the pancreas into the small intestine through the pancreatic duct. (**Side Note**: The pancreas also has an endocrine function, the secretion of insulin and other hormones.)

Pantothenic (PAN-toe-THEN-ick) **Acid**: a B5 vitamin.

Pepsin: a gastric enzyme that hydrolyzes protein. Pepsin is secreted in an inactive form, **pepsinogen**, which is activated by hydrochloric acid in the stomach.

Peptidase: a digestive enzyme that hydrolyzes peptide bonds.

Peptide Bond: a bond that connects the acid end of one amino acid with the amino end of another, forming a link in a protein chain.

Phospholipid (FOS-foe-LIP-id): a compound similar to a triglyceride but having a phosphate group (a phosphorus-containing salt) and choline (or another nitrogen-containing compound) in place of one of the fatty acids.

Phosphorus: a major mineral found mostly in the body's bones and teeth.

Photosynthesis: the process by which green plants make carbohydrates from carbon dioxide and water using the green pigment chlorophyll to trap the sun's energy.

Phytochemicals (FIE-toe-KEM-ih-cals): nonnutrient compounds found in plant-derived foods that have biological activity in the body.

Placenta (plah-SEN-tuh): the organ that develops inside the uterus early in pregnancy, through which the fetus receives nutrients and oxygen and returns carbon dioxide and other waste products to be excreted.

Polypeptide: many (ten or more) amino acids bonded together.

Polyunsaturated Fatty Acid: a fatty acid that lacks four or more hydrogen atoms and has two or more double bonds between carbons.

Potassium: the principal cation within the body's cells; critical to the maintenance of fluid balance, nerve transmissions, and muscle contractions.

Precursors: substances that precede others; with regard to vitamins, compounds that can be converted into active vitamins; also known as **provitamins**.

Prolactin (pro-LAK-tin): a hormone secreted from the anterior pituitary gland that acts on the mammary glands to initiate and sustain milk production.

Protease (PRO-tee-ace): an enzyme that hydrolyzes protein.

Protein Digestibility: a measure of the amount of amino acids absorbed from a given protein intake.

Protein Efficiency Ratio: a measure of protein quality assessed by determining how well a given protein supports weight gain in growing rats; used to establish the protein quality for infant formulas and baby foods.

Proteins: compounds composed of carbon, hydrogen, oxygen, and nitrogen atoms, arranged into amino acids linked in a chain. Some amino acids also contain sulfur atoms.

Puberty: the period in the life in which a person becomes physically capable of reproduction.

Purified Water: water that has been processed through distillation, deionization, or reverse osmosis and meets U.S. Pharmacopoeia standards for medical and research purposes.

Pyloric (pie-LORE-ic) **Sphincter**: the circular muscle that separates the stomach from the small intestine and regulates the flow of partially digested food into the small intestine.

Pyruvate (PIE-roo-vate): pyruvic acid, a 3-carbon compound that plays a key role in energy metabolism.

-R-

Recommended Dietary Allowance (RDA): the average daily amount of a nutrient considered adequate to meet the known nutrient needs of practically all healthy people; a goal for dietary intake by individuals.

Rectum: the muscular terminal part of the intestine, extending from the sigmoid colon to the anus.

Refined: the process by which the coarse parts of a food are removed. When wheat is refined into flour, the bran, germ, and husk are removed, leaving only the endosperm.

Requirement: the lowest continuing intake of a nutrient that will maintain a specified criterion of adequacy.
Riboflavin (RYE-boh-flay-vin): a B2 vitamin.

-S-

Saliva: the secretion of the salivary glands. Its principal enzyme begins carbohydrate digestion.

Salivary Glands: exocrine glands that secrete saliva into the mouth.

Salt: a compound composed a positive ion and a negative ion.

Satiation (say-she-AY-shun): the feeling of satisfaction and fullness that occurs during a meal and halts eating. Satiation determines how much food is consumed during a meal.

Satiety (sah-TIE-eh-tee): the feeling of satisfaction that occurs after a meal and inhibits eating until the next meal. Satiety determines how much time passes between meals.

Saturated Fatty Acid: a fatty acid carrying the maximum possible number of hydrogen atoms. A **saturated fat** is composed of triglycerides in which most of the fatty acids are saturated.

Selenium (se-LEEN-ee-um): a trace mineral.

Set Point: the point at which controls are set (for example, on a thermostat). The set-point theory that relates to the body tends to maintain a certain weight by means of its own internal controls.

Simple Carbohydrates (sugar): monosaccharides and disaccharides.

Small Intestine: a 10-foot length of small-diameter intestine that is the major site of digestion of food and absorption of nutrients.

Sodium: the principal cation in the extracellular fluids of the body; critical to the maintenance of fluid balance, nerve transmissions, and muscle contractions.

Soluble Fibers: indigestible food components that dissolve in water to form a gel. An example is pectin from fruit, which is used to thicken jellies.

Sperm: the male reproductive cell, capable of fertilizing an ovum.

Sphincter (SFINK-ter): a circular muscle surrounding, and able to close, a body opening. Sphincters are found at specific points along the GI tract and regulate the flow of food particles.

Spring Water: water originating from an underground spring or well. It may be carbonated or not. Brand names such as "Spring" or "Pure" do not necessarily mean that the water comes from a spring.

Starches: plant polysaccharides composed of glucose.

Sterols (STARE-ols or STEER-ols): compounds composed of C, H, and O atoms arranged in rings, like those of cholesterol, with any of a variety of side chains attached.

Stomach: a muscular, elastic, saclike, portion of the digestive tract that grinds and churns swallowed food, mixing it with acid and enzymes to form chime.

Stool: waste matter discharged from the colon; also called **feces**.

Stress: any threat to a person's well-being; a demand placed on the body to adapt.

Stroke: an event in which the blood flow to a part of the brain is cut off.

Sucrose (SUE-krose): an artificial sweetener approved for use in the United States.

Supplements: pills, capsules, tablets, liquids, or powders that contain vitamins, minerals, herbs, or amino acids; intended to increase dietary intake of these substances.

-T-

T-cells: lymphocytes that attack antigens. T stands for the thymus gland, where the T-cells are stored for a while.

Testosterone: a steroid hormone from the testicles, or testes.

Thiamin (THIGH-ah-min): a B1 vitamin.

Thyroid-Stimulating Hormone (TSH): a hormone secreted by the pituitary that stimulates the thyroid gland to secrete its hormones— thyroxine and triiodothyronine.

Toxicity: the ability of a substance to harm living organisms. All substances are toxic if high enough concentrations are used.

Trace Minerals: essential mineral nutrients found in the human body in amounts smaller than 5 g; sometimes called microminerals.

***Trans*-fatty Acids**: fatty acids with an unusual configuration around the double bond.

Triglycerides (try-GLISS-er-rides): the chief form of fat in the diet and the major storage form of fat in the body.

Tripeptide: three amino acids bonded together.

Type I Diabetes: the less common type of diabetes in which the person produces no insulin at all.

Type II Diabetes: the more common type of diabetes in which the fat cells resist insulin.

-U-

Umbilical (um-BILL-ih-cul) **Cord**: the cordlike structure through which the fetus's veins and arteries reach the placenta; the route of nourishment and oxygen to the fetus and the route of waste disposal from the fetus.

Underweight: body weight below some standard of acceptable weight that is usually defined in relation to height (such as BMI).

Unsaturated Fatty Acid: a fatty acid that lacks hydrogen atom and has at least one double bond between carbons (includes monounsaturated and polyunsaturated fatty acids). An **unsaturated fat** is composed of triglycerides in which most of the fatty acids are unsaturated.

Urea (you-REE-uh): the principal nitrogen-excretion product of metabolism. Two ammonia fragments are combined with carbon dioxide to form urea.

Uterus (YOU-ter-us): the muscular organ within which the infant develops before birth.

-V-

Variety (dietary): eating a wide selection of foods within and among the major food groups.

Vegetarians: a general term used to describe people who exclude meat, poultry, fish, or other animal-derived foods from their diets.

Vitamin A: all naturally occurring compounds with the biological activity of retinol (RET-ih-nol), the alcohol form of vitamin A

Vitamins: organic, essential nutrients required in small amounts by the body for health.

VLDL (Very-low-density lipoprotein): the type of lipoprotein made primarily by liver cells to transport lipids to various tissues in the body; composed primarily of triglycerides.

-W-

Water Balance: the balance between water intake and output (losses).

Water Intoxication: the rare condition in which the body water contents are too high.

Weight Training: the use of free weights or weight machines to provide resistance for developing muscle strength and endurance. A person's own body weight may also provide resistance as when a person does push-ups, pull-ups, or abdominal crunches.

Whole Grain: a grain milled in its entirety (all but the husk), not refined.

-Y-

Yogurt: milk fermented by specific bacterial cultures.

SUBJECT INDEX

A

acetyl CoA (acetyl coenzyme A), 14–17, 18–19

acid-base balance, 108–9

acids

    fatty, 7, 12, 18–19, 67–70, 76–77

    folic, 123, 125

    keto, 17

    lactic, 15

    linoleic, 76

    linolenic, 76–77

    pantothenic, 92

    trans-fatty, 8–9, 69–70, 79–80

    See also amino acids

activities, 182–83, 199, 203–4

adenosine triphosphate (ATP), 13

adequate intake (AI), 20–23

ADH (antidiuretic hormone), 106

adipose tissues, 77–78

adolescents, 152–56, 160–61, 199

F

H

I

infants, 135–36, 139–42, 199

infections, 62

insulin, 35–36

interstitial fluid, 103

intestines, 31–32, 48, 72–73

intolerances, 151

intracellular fluid, 103

iodine, 10, 99

iron

    adults and, 170

    childhood and, 146

    infants and, 141

    pregnancy and, 123–26, 137

    as trace minerals, 10, 99–100

J

joint disorders, proteins and, 7

K

keto acid, 17

ketone bodies, 34

ketosis, 34

RECIPE INDEX

www.ingramcontent.com/pod-product-compliance
Lightning Source LLC
Chambersburg PA
CBHW060447290526
45791CB00001B/15